Emergencies at High Altitude A Ready Reckoner for Healthcare Workers

Contributors

Brig Vinay Kumar Maurya
Consultant (Radiology),
Brig Med, 14 Corps

Brig Rajan Kapoor, VSM
Consultant (Internal Medicine) & Haematologist
Commandant, 153 General Hospital

Col Ravdeep Singh Sohal
Senior Advisor (Surgery) & CTVS surgeon
Senior registrar & OC troops, 153 General Hospital

Maj Ravi Kumar
Medical Specialist (Internal Medicine)
153 General Hospital

Editor

Maj Ravi Kumar
Medical Specialist (Internal Medicine)
153 General Hospital

notionpress.com

INDIA · SINGAPORE · MALAYSIA

ISBN
Paperback 979-8-90560-162-0
Hardcase 979-8-90560-163-7

EMERGENCIES AT HIGH ALTITUDE
A READY RECKONER FOR HEALTHCARE WORKERS

NON-DISCLOSURE

Medical knowledge and its practice change constantly. This book is designed to provide accurate and authoritative information about the subject matter in question. However, readers are advised to check the most current information available on procedures included and check information from the manufacturer of each product to be administered to verify the recommended dose, formula, method, duration of administration, adverse effects, and contraindications. It is the responsibility of the practitioner to take all appropriate safety precautions. Neither the publisher nor the author/ editors assume any liability for any injury and/or damage to persons or property arising from or related to the use of the material in this book.

Every effort has been made where necessary to contact holders of copyright to obtain permission to reproduce copyright material. If any has been inadvertently overlooked, the publisher will be pleased to make the necessary arrangements at the first opportunity. This book is sold on the understanding that the publisher is not engaged in providing professional medical services. If such advice or services are required, the services of a competent medical professional should be sought.

E-mail : 153gh@gmail.com

This book is dedicated to the brave soldiers of the Indian Army who serve with unwavering courage and endurance in the formidable heights of the Himalayas, and to all the dedicated soldiers whose commitment to excellence, professionalism, and compassion exemplifies the finest traditions of the Armed Forces Medical Services.

It stands as a tribute to all health care workers posted to high-altitude areas - who provide care under extreme conditions, transform hardship into learning, and uphold the sacred duty of preserving the health and lives of those who guard our nation's frontiers.

This work also honours the spirit of knowledge-sharing -to guide and educate those newly inducted into high-altitude service, to assist practitioners who seldom encounter such unique challenges, and to continue the legacy of 153 General Hospital as a beacon of clinical excellence, research, and teaching in the realm of high-altitude medicine.

लेफ्टिनेंट जनरल हितेश भल्ला, यू वाई एस एम, एस सी**, एस एम, वी एस एम
जनरल ऑफिसर कमांडिंग एवं
कर्नल ऑफ दि मराठा एल आई

*Lt Gen Hitesh Bhalla, UYSM, SC**, SM, VSM*

General Officer Commanding &
Colonel of The MARATHA LI

मुख्यालय १४ कोर
पिन - ९०८५१४
द्वारा ५६ ए पी ओ
Headquarters 14 Corps
PIN - 908514
C/o 56 APO

कर्त्तव्य, मान, साहस
DUTY, HONOUR, COURAGE

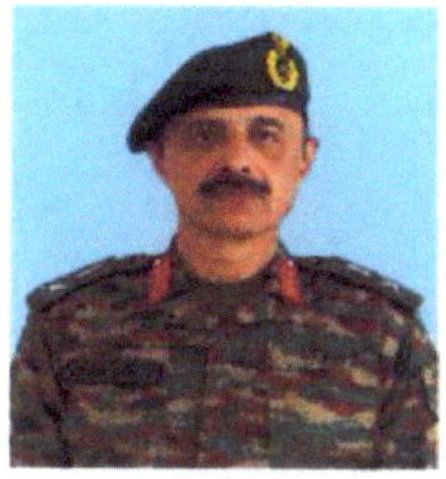

Foreword

1. It gives me immense satisfaction to know that the book titled "***Emergencies at High Altitude-A Ready Reckoner for Health Care Workers***" has been developed as a practical guide for medical personnel serving in high-altitude and operationally demanding environments by 153 General Hospital under the aegis of HQ, 14 Corps (Medical Branch).

2. The high-altitude terrain presents unique medical and logistical challenges where timely recognition, swift decision-making, and efficient management are essential. Healthcare workers deployed in such areas often function under challenging climatic, geographical, and resource constraint conditions while providing critical medical support to troops and civilians alike. The strength of this handbook lies in its simplicity and practicality. The use of concise tables, algorithms, checklists, and protocol-based approaches makes it an effective field reference for rapid assessment and emergency management in real-world situations.

3. I compliment the authors and contributors for their dedicated effort in creating a compact, operationally relevant, and clinically useful resource tailored to the requirements of healthcare workers in high-altitude areas. Such initiatives significantly contribute toward strengthening medical preparedness, improving emergency response capability, and enhancing healthcare delivery in forward and remote locations.

4. I am confident that this publication will serve as a valuable companion for medical officers, nursing staff, paramedics, and all healthcare personnel working in extreme environments. I extend my best wishes to the entire team for this commendable academic contribution and wish the publication great success.

Station: Leh

Date: 01 Jun 2026

Hitesh Bhalla
Lt Gen
GOC, 14 Corps

ब्रिगेडियर विनय कुमार मौर्य
ब्रिग मेड
Brig Vinay Kumar Maurya
Brig Med
Tele No. : 3279 (O)
2773 (R)

मुख्यालय 14 कोर
पिन–908514
द्वारा 56 ए पी ओ
Headquarters 14 Corps
Pin - 908514
C/o 56 APO

सर्वे सन्तु निराभया

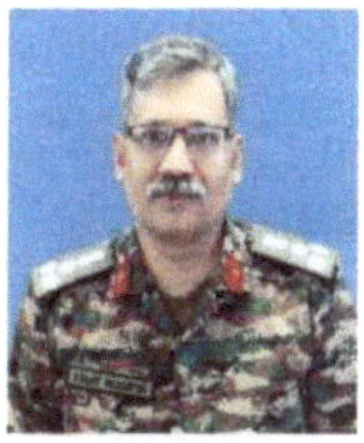

Preface

1. High-altitude emergencies demand rapid recognition, prompt decision-making, and protocol-based management. In remote and resource-limited terrains, healthcare workers often function under extreme environmental and operational constraints where timely intervention becomes critical for survival.

2. **"Emergencies at High Altitude – A Ready Reckoner for Health Care Workers"** has been designed as a simple, practical, and field-oriented handbook focusing on emergency assessment and immediate management in high-altitude areas. The table-based and algorithmic approach adopted in this book makes it easy to understand, quick to revise, and practical to apply during real-time emergencies. The book successfully simplifies important high-altitude medical conditions and operational emergencies into concise flowcharts, checklists, and management pathways for use by medical officers, nursing staff, paramedics, and frontline healthcare workers.

3. I commend the authors and contributors for their efforts in developing a clinically relevant and operationally useful guide tailored for challenging high-altitude environments. Such academic initiatives strengthen preparedness, improve response capability, and support quality healthcare delivery in remote operational areas.

4. I am confident that this handbook will serve as a valuable companion for healthcare personnel working in high-altitude regions and will contribute meaningfully toward improving emergency care and patient outcomes. I extend my best wishes to the entire team for this commendable academic endeavour.

Station: Leh

Date : 30 May 26

Vinay Kumar Maurya
Brig
Brig (Med), 14 Corps

INDEX

CHAPTER 1
INITIAL ASSESSMENT & STABILIZATION

"The first 10 minutes determine survival."

At high altitude, critically ill patients deteriorate rapidly because of hypobaric hypoxia, delayed evacuation, cold stress, and limited resources. Early recognition and aggressive stabilization are essential.

The primary goals are:

- *Stabilize airway, breathing, and circulation*
- *Recognize HAPE/HACE early*
- *Initiate timely CASEVAC*

Severe respiratory failure
Recurrent seizures
Airway protection failure
Severe HACE with altered sensorium

1. ABCDE APPROACH

The ABCDE approach provides a structured method to assess and stabilize all emergencies at high altitude.

A – AIRWAY

Rapid Assessment

Look for:

- *Ability to speak*
- *Snoring/gurgling*
- *Secretions/vomitus, Stridor*
- *Facial trauma*
- *Reduced consciousness*

nask	**L/min**	**ıte distress**

Immediate Actions

Airway Algorithm

Assess airway
↓
Patent?

YES — *Monitor Oxygen*
NO — *Open airway & Suction*
↓
Improved?

YES — *Monitoring*
NO — *OPA/NPA*
↓
Need definitive airway?
↓
Intubate

B – BREATHING

Breathing abnormalities are the most common life-threatening problems at high altitude.

Rapid Assessment

Assess:

- *Respiratory rate, SpO_2, Work of breathing*
- *Accessory muscle use, Crepitations/wheeze*
- *Cyanosis, Chest expansion*

Severe HAPE/HACE	**est achievable**

Breathing Algorithm

Breathless patient
↓
Check S... RR
↓
Severe ...

YES — NO

NRBM oxygen — Nasal oxygen

IV acce...
↓
Crackles present?

YES — NO

Consider HAPE — Evaluate other causes
↓
Persistent hypoxia?
↓
HFNC/NIV → Intubation if worsening

monia	Fever + focal signs

High-R...

$SpO_2 < 80\%$, $RR > 30/min$, Silent chest

Severe cyanosis, Exhaustion, Altered sensorium

C – CIRCULATION

Circulatory instability worsens rapidly at altitude because hypoxia impairs tissue perfusion.

Rapid Assessment

Check: Pulse, BP, Capillary refill, Skin temperature, Peripheral perfusion, Jugular venous pressure, Urine output

Common Causes of Shock

: shock	Fever + hypotension

Red Flag Signs

Ataxia

Altered behaviour

Seizures

Immediate Stabilization

- ***IV Access:*** *Two large-bore IV cannulas*
- ***Monitoring:*** ECG, BP, Urine output
- ***Fluid Therapy:*** *Use crystalloids cautiously (Avoid aggressive fluids in HAPE)*
- ***Vasopressor Support:*** *If hypotension persists then Noradrenaline preferred (0.05–1 mcg/kg/min IV infusion)*

Circulation Algorithm

Hypotension/shock
↓
IV acce...
↓
Signs of fluid loss?

YES — NO

Fluid bo...

10–20...
↓
MAP improving?

YES — NO

Continue monitoring — Start vasopressor + urgent referral

Severe breathlessness at rest

$SpO_2 < 80\%$ despite oxygen

Confusion/ataxia, Cyanosis

Pulmonary edema signs

$RR > 30/min$, $GCS < 13$

Recurrent vomiting with neurological symptoms

D – DISABILITY

Neurological deterioration at altitude may indicate HACE, stroke, hypoglycaemia, or seizures.

Rapid Assessment

Assess: GCS, Pupils, Limb weakness, Confusion, Ataxia, Speech, Blood glucose

Immediate Actions

Check glucose immediately: *Treat hypoglycaemia promptly*

Suspected HACE: *Oxygen immediately & Dexamethasone 8 mg IV stat*

Seizure Management: Lorazepam *(4 mg IV) OR* **Midazolam** *(5–10 mg IV/IM)*

E – EXPOSURE

Complete examination is essential to avoid missing trauma, frostbite, or hypothermia.

Assess For

- *Hypothermia, Frostbite, Trauma, bleeding, Rash/infection*

Prevent Heat Loss

Important Measures

- *Remove wet clothing, warm blankets, warm IV fluids if possible, avoid prolonged exposure*

2. OXYGEN THERAPY

Golden Rule: *"Hypoxia worsens every emergency at high altitude."*

Oxygen is the single most important intervention in critically ill patients at altitude.

Principles

Start oxygen early if:

- *SpO_2 low, Breathlessness present, HAPE/HACE suspected, shock present or altered sensorium present*

Oxygen Escalation Strategy

Hypoxia detected
↓
Nasal prongs

YES ***NO***

Continue monitoring | *Face mask/NRBM*
↓
Persistent hypoxia?
↓
HFNC/NIV
↓
Failure?
↓
Intubation

3. MONITORING

Continuous monitoring prevents delayed deterioration.

Essential Monitoring Parameters

	ıtinuous
ırature	ıular

→

ling SpO_2
ing RR
rsening confusion

4. CASEVAC PRINCIPLES

CASEVAC = Treatment + Transport

Evacuation should never be delayed in critically ill patie

Before

Stabiliz

- Airway secure, Oxygen ongoing
- IV access established, Monitoring attached

Indications for Immediate CASEVAC

- **Suspected HACE or Severe HAPE**
- **Respiratory failure**
- **Need for ventilatory support**
- **ACS/STEMI or Polytrauma**
- **Recurrent seizures**

During Transport

Maintain:

- Oxygen therapy, Warmth hemodynamic monitoring, communication with receiving center

CASEVAC Algorithm

Critically ill patient

↓

Stabiliz

↓

Need higher center care?

YES **NO**

Prepare

↓

Secure

↓

Monitor during transport

↓

Early handover to receiving center

Shock
ACS/STEMI
Stroke
Respiratory failure
Active seizures
Severe trauma

5. EMERGENCY TRIAGE

Triage Categories

V	llness	ine care
(	ivable/no signs of life	ative/expectant

Operational Pearls

- "Confusion at altitude is HACE until proven otherwise."
- "Breathlessness with crackles is HAPE until proven otherwise."
- "Early oxygen and early descent save lives."
- "The sickest patients deteriorate fastest during delayed evacuation."

Practic

at hypoxia early ssess frequently pect HAPE/HACE early	Delay oxygen therapy & overload fluids in HAPE Ignore confusion at altitude Delay evacuation in severe illness

tinalli JE, Ma OJ, Yealy DM, et al. Tintinalli's Emergency Medicine: A Comprehensive Study Guide. 9th ed. New McGraw-Hill; 2020.
ks AM, Auerbach PS, Freer L, et al. Wilderness Medical Society Clinical Practice Guidelines for the Prevention reatment of Acute Altitude Illness. Wilderness Environ Med. 2019;30(4 Suppl):S3–S18.

CHAPTER 1 INITIAL ASSESSMENT & STABILIZATION

1. DEFINITION

Rapid identification and immediate management of life-threatening illness or injury in high-altitude environments to prevent deterioration and prepare for safe evacuation.

2. WHY DANGEROUS AT HIGH ALTITUDE

- Reduced oxygen → rapid hypoxia
- Lower physiological reserve
- Minor illness can deteriorate quickly
- Cold, dehydration, exertion worsen instability
- Delayed evacuation increases mortality

3. RED FLAG SIGNS

- SpO_2 < 80% despite oxygen
- Severe breathlessness at rest
- Altered sensorium / confusion
- Ataxia / unable to walk
- Cyanosis
- Hypotension / shock
- Chest pain suggestive of ACS / PE
- Seizures
- RR > 30/min
- GCS < 13
- Persistent vomiting with neurological symptoms
- Pulmonary edema signs
- Hemodynamic instability

4. RAPID ASSESSMENT

A. KEY HISTORY

- Recent ascent?
- Altitude reached?
- Rate of ascent?
- Breathlessness?
- Headache / ataxia / confusion?
- Fever / cough?
- Chest pain / palpitations?
- Trauma / fall?
- Cold exposure?

B. RAPID EXAMINATION

- **Airway:** Patent? Secretions? Gurgling / snoring?
- **Breathing:** RR, SpO_2, accessory muscle use, crackles / wheeze?
- **Circulation:** Pulse, BP, capillary refill, perfusion?
- **Disability:** GCS, pupils, confusion, ataxia, seizures?
- **Exposure:** Hypothermia, trauma, frostbite, wounds?

C. MONITORING

- SpO_2
- ECG
- BP (NIBP/IBP)
- RR
- Temperature
- Urine output
- Level of consciousness
- Blood glucose

D. TARGETS

- SpO_2 > 90%
- MAP > 65 mmHg
- RR < 24/min
- Urine output > 0.5 mL/kg/hr
- Temp > 35°C

5. IMMEDIATE STABILIZATION (ABCDE APPROACH)

A – AIRWAY

- Check patency
- Jaw thrust / chin lift
- Suction if needed
- DPA/NPA if required
- Intubate if: GCS ≤ 8, severe resp failure, recurrent seizures

B – BREATHING

- Start oxygen immediately
- Use appropriate device (see right)
- Assist ventilation if inadequate
- Consider HFNC / NIV if available
- Intubate if failing oxygenation/ventilation

C – CIRCULATION

- IV access × 2 (large bore)
- Monitor BP, HR, ECG
- Assess perfusion, cap refill
- Treat hypotension / shock
- Avoid fluid overload in HAPE

D – DISABILITY

- Check GCS, pupils, BSL
- Treat seizures promptly
- Consider HACE / stroke
- Protect airway if GCS ≤ 8

E – EXPOSURE

- Expose fully, look for injuries
- Prevent heat loss
- Warm blankets / fluids
- Remove wet clothing

OXYGEN STRATEGY

Condition	Device
Mild hypoxia	Nasal prongs (2–6 L/min)
Moderate distress	Face mask (6–10 L/min)
Severe hypoxia	NRBM (10–15 L/min)
Persistent failure	HFNC / NIV
Impending collapse	Intubation

SHOCK ACTION

- Crystalloid bolus 10–20 mL/kg
- Reassess
- Start vasopressor if MAP < 65 mmHg after fluids

SEIZURE MANAGEMENT

Lorazepam 4 mg IV OR
Midazolam 5–10 mg IM/IV

6. DIAGNOSTIC ALGORITHM

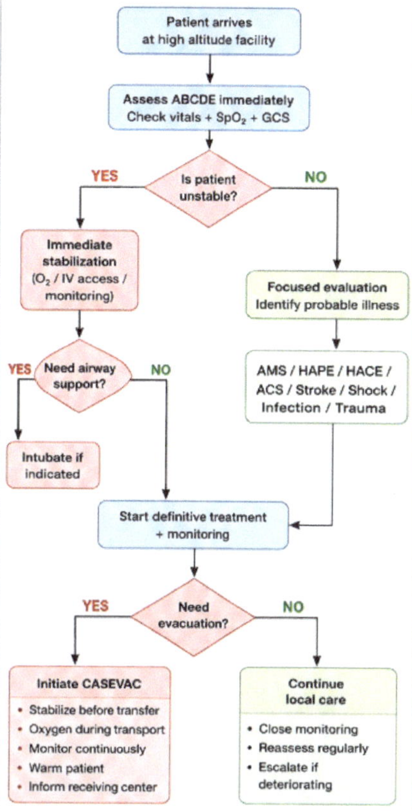

7. TREATMENT PROTOCOL (INITIAL BUNDLE)

1. **Oxygen** – Start immediately
2. **Monitoring** – SpO_2, ECG, BP, RR, Temp, Urine output
3. **IV Access** – Two large-bore cannulas
4. **Point-of-Care Tests** – BSL, ECG, ABG (if available)
5. **Identify & Treat Reversible Causes**

CAUSE	IMMEDIATE ACTION
Hypoglycemia	IV dextrose
HAPE	Oxygen + Nifedipine
HACE	Dexamethasone
Shock	Fluids / Vasopressors
ACS / STEMI	STEMI protocol
Seizure	Benzodiazepines
Sepsis	Antibiotics + Fluids

EMERGENCY DRUG BOX (ADULT)

Drug	Dose	Indication
Dexamethasone	8 mg IV stat then 4 mg 6-hrly	HACE
Nifedipine SR	30 mg PO	HAPE
Lorazepam	4 mg IV	Seizures
Midazolam	5–10 mg IM/IV	Seizures
Noradrenaline	0.05–1 mcg/kg/min	Shock
Adrenaline	1 mg IV/IO	Cardiac arrest
Amiodarone	300 mg IV bolus	VF/pVT

8. EVACUATION CRITERIA

- Severe hypoxia despite oxygen
- HAPE (suspected / confirmed)
- HACE (suspected / confirmed)
- Respiratory failure / need for ventilatory support
- Stroke / focal neurological deficit
- Persistent shock
- ACS / STEMI
- Recurrent seizures
- Polytrauma
- Deteriorating consciousness

9. PRACTICAL PEARLS

DO

- ✔ Treat hypoxia early
- ✔ Reassess frequently
- ✔ Keep patient warm
- ✔ Think HAPE / HACE in any deteriorating patient
- ✔ Use pulse oximetry serially
- ✔ Evacuate early rather than late

DO NOT

- ✖ Overload fluids in breathless patients
- ✖ Ignore altered behavior / confusion
- ✖ Delay oxygen therapy
- ✖ Miss hypoglycemia
- ✖ Delay evacuation in neurological symptoms

OPERATIONAL PEARLS

- "Confusion at altitude is HACE until proven otherwise."
- "Breathlessness with crackles at altitude is HAPE until proven otherwise."
- "Hypoxia worsens every emergency at altitude."
- "Early oxygen and early descent save lives."

ASSESS RAPIDLY • STABILIZE EARLY • EVACUATE SAFELY • SAVE LIVES

CHAPTER 2
ACUTE MOUNTAIN SICKNESS (AMS)

"Headache at altitude is AMS until proven otherwise."

Acute Mountain Sickness (AMS) is the commonest altitude-related illness and usually develops after rapid ascent above 2,500 meters. Early recognition is critical because AMS may progress to High-Altitude Cerebral Edema (HACE), which is life-threatening.

1. RECOGNITION

Definition: *AMS is a syndrome of headache with other symptoms occurring after recent ascent to high altitude in a previously unacclimatized individual. Typical onset: 6–24 hours after ascent, usually within first 1–2 days*

Why AMS Occurs at High Altitude

Reduced atmospheric oxygen causes:

- *Hypobaric hypoxia& cerebral vasodilation*
- *Mild cerebral edema*
- *Fluid shifts & Sleep disturbances*

isk increases with:
apid ascent, Overexertion
oor acclimatization
evious AMS history

Common Symptoms

che & Fatigue	ommon

adache
Confusion or decreasing consciousness
Breathlessness at rest or cyanosis
hese suggest progression to:

AMS Recognition Algorithm

Recent ascent > 2500 m
↓
Headache present?

YES
Assess symptoms *AMS unlikely*
(fatigue/nausea/dizziness/sleep disturbance)
↓
Symptoms mild?

Severe fatigue, SpO_2 markedly low

YES **NO**
Likely AMS *Evaluate for severe AMS/HACE*

2. LAKE LOUISE SCORE (LLS)

Lake Louise Scoring System is the standard bedside tool for diagnosing AMS.
Diagnostic Criteria for AMS

- **Recent ascent to altitude + Headache is present + Total LLS ≥ 3**

3–5	**Mild AMS**

2018 Revised Lake Louise Scoring System (Current Standard in 2026)

che	None	Mild headache	Moderate headache	e/incapacitating che
ess / headedness	None	Mild	Moderate	e/incapacitating ess

*Important Update: **Sleep disturbance was removed from the scoring system in the 2018 revision because it poorly correlated with true AMS.***

Importc
AMS

Symptoms worsening
Ataxia develops
Confusion appears

3. IMMEDIATE MANAGEMENT

Goals of Treatment

- *Improve oxygenation*
- *Prevent progression to HACE/HAPE*
- *Relieve symptoms*
- *Stop further ascent & consider descent if worsening*

Immediate Steps for Initial Stabilization

- ***Stop further ascent** (This is the single most important step)*
- ***Rest** (Avoid exertion)*
- ***Oxygen Therapy***
- ***Give oxygen if:** Moderate/severe AMS, SpO_2 low, Symptoms worsening, Target: $SpO_2 > 90\%$*
- ***Symptomatic Treatment***
- ***Headache: Paracetamol** (500–1000 mg PO) **OR Ibuprofen** (400–600 mg PO)*
- ***Nausea/Vomiting: Ondansetron** (4 mg IV/PO)*

Specific Therapy

Acetazolamide
***Mechanism:** Improves acclimatization & Stimulates ventilation*
***Treatment Dose:** 250 mg PO twice daily*
Important Notes

- *Continue for 24–48 hrs after symptom resolution & **avoid in severe sulfa allergy***

Dexamethasone
***Used for:** Severe AMS, Suspected progression to HACE*
***Dose:** 8 mg IV/PO stat THEN 4 mg every 6 hours*

AMS Treatment Algorithm

Diagnosed AMS
↓
Stop ascent immediately
↓
Mild symptoms?

YES	NO
Rest + fluids	Oxygen
Analgesics	Acetazolamide
Observation	Dexamethasone if severe
↓	↓
Improving?	Signs of HACE/HAPE?

YES	NO	YES	NO
Observe	Descent	Immediate descent	Continue treatment

Drug Box

Drug	Dose	Purpose
Paracetamol	500–1000 mg	Headache

4. PREVENTION

Golden Rule: *"Prevention is better than evacuation."*

Safe Ascent Principles

Above 3000 m:

- *Increase sleeping altitude gradually & avoid rapid ascent*

Recommended Ascent

General Preventive Measures

Adequate hydration, avoid alcohol/sedatives, avoid overexertion, light meals initially, gradual acclimatization

Acetazolamide Prophylaxis

Indications: *Previous AMS history, rapid ascent unavoidable, high-risk individuals*

- **Dose:** *125 mg PO twice daily*
- **Start:** *24 hours before ascent and* **continue** *till 48 hours after highest altitude reached*

Prevention Algorithm

Planning ascent > 2500 m

↓

Previous AMS history?

YES	**NO**
Acetazolamide prophylaxis	*Gradual ascent + hydration*

↓

Avoid rapid ascent/exertion

↓

Monitor for symptoms daily

↓

YES	**NO**
Stop ascent *Evaluate AMS*	*Continue ascent*

Practic

end gradually & treat headache early *p ascent if symptoms appear*	*T* *re headache at altitude* *tinue ascent with symptoms*

Operational Pearls

- *"The best treatment for AMS is stopping ascent."*
- *"AMS progression can be rapid at extreme altitude."*
- *"Ataxia is never a feature of simple AMS & Persistent headache + confusion = HACE until proven otherwise."*

snyat B, Murdoch DR. High-altitude illness. Lancet. 2003;361(9373):1967-1974.

cs AM, Swenson ER, Bärtsch P. Acute high-altitude sickness. Eur Respir Rev. 2017;26(143):160096.

CHAPTER 2: ACUTE MOUNTAIN SICKNESS (AMS)

AMS RECOGNITION & MANAGEMENT ALGORITHM

RECENT ASCENT > 2500 m
Patient develops **HEADACHE**

↓

Assess associated symptoms
Fatigue / Nausea / Dizziness / Poor sleep

↓

Apply LAKE LOUISE SCORE
(Score ≥ 3 ?)

- **YES** → **LIKELY AMS** → **Assess severity** → **Any RED FLAG signs?** Ataxia / Confusion / Severe hypoxia / Breathlessness at rest / Cyanosis
  - **YES** → **SUSPECT HACE / HAPE**
    - Immediate oxygen
    - Dexamethasone
    - Urgent descent
    - CASEVAC if needed
    - Continuous monitoring

    → Continue observation / Avoid further ascent
  - **NO** → **MILD – MODERATE AMS**
    - Stop further ascent
    - Rest
    - Oral fluids
    - Analgesics
    - Acetazolamide

    → **Reassess after 12–24 hrs** → **Symptoms improving?**
    - **YES** → **Continue observation** / Avoid further ascent
    - **NO** → **DESCEND** / Reassess for HACE / HAPE
- **NO** → **AMS UNLIKELY** / Evaluate other causes

LAKE LOUISE SCORING SYSTEM

Score each symptom: 0 = None, 1 = Mild, 2 = Moderate, 3 = Severe

Symptom	0	1	2	3
Headache	None	Mild	Moderate	Severe
GI symptoms (nausea/vomiting)	None	Poor appetite	Nausea	Vomiting
Fatigue / Weakness	None	Mild	Moderate	Severe
Dizziness / Lightheadedness	None	Mild	Moderate	Severe
Sleep disturbance	Normal	Mild disturbance	Frequent waking	Severe insomnia

INTERPRETATION

- 0 – 2 : No AMS
- 3 – 5 : Mild AMS
- ≥ 6 : Severe AMS

RED FLAG SIGNS (Think HACE / HAPE)

- Ataxia / unable to walk straight
- Confusion / altered behavior
- Severe persistent headache
- Persistent vomiting
- Breathlessness at rest
- SpO_2 < 80% / severe hypoxia
- Cyanosis
- Decreasing level of consciousness

KEY MANAGEMENT PRINCIPLES

- **STOP** further ascent
- **OXYGEN** early if moderate/severe or hypoxic
- **REST** and avoid exertion
- **HYDRATE** adequately
- **DESCEND** if worsening or red flags develop

PREVENTION ALGORITHM

Planning ascent > 2500 m → **Previous AMS history?**

- **YES** → **High-risk ascent?** → **Start Acetazolamide** 125 mg twice daily (Start 24 h before ascent)
- **NO** → **Gradual ascent**
  - Hydration
  - Avoid overexertion
  - Avoid alcohol / sedatives

↓

Ascend gradually
Increase sleeping altitude by ≤ 500 m/day above 3000 m
Add rest day every 3–4 days

↓

Daily symptom monitoring → **Symptoms develop?**

- **YES** → **Stop ascent** / Evaluate for AMS / Treat accordingly
- **NO** → **Continue ascent** / Monitor daily

SEVERE AMS / HACE ESCALATION ALGORITHM

AMS patient Deteriorating

↓

Check for:

- Ataxia
- Confusion
- Persistent vomiting
- Severe headache
- Reduced consciousness
- Focal neurological deficit

↓

Any present?

- **YES** → **TREAT AS HACE**
  - High-flow oxygen
  - Dexamethasone 8 mg IV stat then 4 mg IV 6 hourly
  - Prepare IMMEDIATE DESCENT
  - CASEVAC urgently

  → **Monitor continuously** Airway, SpO_2, GCS, Vitals
- **NO** → **Continue AMS treatment**
  - Rest
  - Oxygen if needed
  - Acetazolamide
  - Analgesics
  - Reassess closely

DRUG DOSES (ADULT)

Acetazolamide (Treatment)	250 mg PO twice daily
Acetazolamide (Prevention)	125 mg PO twice daily
Dexamethasone	8 mg IV stat then 4 mg IV every 6 hourly
Paracetamol	500–1000 mg PO every 6–8 hourly
Ibuprofen	400–600 mg PO every 8 hourly
Ondansetron	4 mg IV/PO every 8 hourly

EARLY RECOGNITION • EARLY TREATMENT • EARLY DESCENT • SAVE LIVES

CHAPTER 3
HIGH-ALTITUDE PULMONARY EDEMA (HAPE)

"Breathlessness at altitude is HAPE until proven otherwise."

High-Altitude Pulmonary Edema (HAPE) is a potentially fatal, non-cardiogenic pulmonary edema that develops after ascent to high altitude, usually above 2500 m. Early recognition, oxygen therapy, and descent are life-saving.

1. RECOGNITION

Definition: *HAPE is a hypoxia-induced pulmonary edema caused by exaggerated pulmonary vasoconstriction and increased pulmonary artery pressure leading to alveolar fluid leakage.*

Typical onset:

-

Why HAPE Occurs at High Altitude

Hypoxia causes:

- *Pulmonary vasoconstriction & elevated pulmonary artery pressure*
- *Cc*
- *Im*

Breathlessness at rest
SpO_2 < 85% or RR > 30/min
Severe cyanosis, Frothy sputum

Hemodynamic instability

Typical Symptoms

ie	*feature*
ed exercise tolerance	*ion*

Fine-to-coarse crackles
Cyanosis, Pink frothy sputum
Respiratory distress, Exhaustion

Important Clinical Point: *"Absence of fever in a breathless patient at altitude strongly suggests HAPE."*

Recognition Algorithm

Recent ascent >2500 m
↓
Breathlessness develops
↓
Check:
SpO_2 + RR + HR + auscultation
↓
Crackles present?

YES	NO
Suspect HAPE	Evaluate other causes

↓
Severe hypoxia?

YES	NO
Immediate oxygen + urgent descent	Start treatment Monitor closely

k Factors	
ıpid ascent	**important**
igh sleeping altitude	**ısed incidence**

2. DIFFERENTIAL DIAGNOSIS

Important Conditions Mimicking HAPE

Condition	Key Features	Features Against HAPE
Pneumonia	Fever, productive cough	Focal consolidation
Pulmonary embolism	Sudden chest pain	Risk factors for thrombosis
ACS/LV failure	Cardiac history	Raised JVP, edema
COPD/Asthma	Wheeze	Prior history
Viral infection	URI symptoms	Mild hypoxia

HAPE vs Pneumonia

Feature	HAPE	Pneumonia
Fever	Usually absent	Common
Crackles	Bilateral	Often focal
Response to oxygen	Dramatic	Partial
Response to descent	Rapid	Variable
Sputum	Frothy	Purulent

Important Monitoring

Parameter	Frequency
SpO_2	Continuous
RR, HR & BP	Hourly
Urine output	4 hourly
Mental status	Serial

Investigations

Bedside
Pulse oximetry: Markedly low saturation
Chest auscultation: Bilateral crackles
ECG: Sinus tachycardia common
Chest X-ray
Typical findings:

- Patchy bilateral infiltrates
- Perihilar opacities, non-cardiogenic pattern

HAPE vs Cardiogenic Pulmonary Edema

Feature	HAPE	Cardiogenic Edema
History	Usually absent	Common
Pedal edema	Rare	Common
JVP	Usually normal	Elevated
Age	Younger patients	Older/comorbid
Trigger	Altitude ascent	Cardiac disease

3. OXYGEN & DRUG THERAPY

GOLDEN RULE

"Oxygen and descent are the definitive treatments for HAPE."

A. OXYGEN THERAPY

Start Immediately: All suspected HAPE patients require oxygen.

Oxygen Targets

Severity	Target
Mild HAPE	$SpO_2 > 90\%$
Severe HAPE	Highest achievable

Oxygen Delivery Devices

Device	Flow Rate	Use
Nasal prongs	2–6 L/min	Mild cases
Face mask	6–10 L/min	Moderate distress
NRBM	10–15 L/min	Severe hypoxia
HFNC	High flow	Persistent hypoxia
NIV	CPAP/BiPAP	Severe distress
Intubation	–	Respiratory failure

Positioning
Keep patient: Sitting upright, warm, resting
Avoid: Exertion and further ascent

B. DRUG THERAPY

Nifedipine (First-line Drug)
Mechanism

- Pulmonary vasodilation, & reduces pulmonary artery pressure

Dose: Sustained-release nifedipine (30 mg PO every 12 hourly) OR **Immediate-release nifedipine** (10 mg PO stat THEN 20 mg SR after stabilization)

Importc

Monitor BP carefully, avoid severe hypotension, continue until descent/improvement

Alternative Drug

Sildenafil: Used if nifedipine unavailable/intolerant.

Dose: 50 mg PO every 8 hours

Supportive Therapy

- **Hydration:** Maintain hydration cautiously
- **Avoid Fluid Overload:** Excess fluids worsen pulmonary edema.
- **Diuretics: Routine use NOT recommended.** Use only if:
  - Fluid overload evident or cardiac failure suspected [**Furosemide** (20–40 mg IV cautiously)]

Morphine

May help severe distress/anxiety (2–4 mg IV cautiously)

Monitor: Respiratory depression

Expected Response

Improvement usually occurs within:

- 30–60 minutes of oxygen
- Several hours after treatment/descent

Morphine	**2–4 mg IV**	**Severe distress**

4. HAPE ALGORITHM

Patient at altitude with breathlessness

↓

Check SpO_2 + RR + auscultation

↓

Crackles + severe hypoxia?

YES — NO

Suspect HAPE — Evaluate other causes

↓

Start high-flow oxygen immediately, Sit upright + keep warm

Restrict exertion

↓

Start ni

↓

YES — NO

Continue treatment — Escalate oxygen

Avoid ascent — HFNC/NIV

Plan descent — Prepare CASEVAC/ Consider ICU

Severe HAPE Algorithm

Severe HAPE suspected

SpO_2 <ξ

High-fl

↓

Nifedipine + continuous monitoring

↓

Need ventilatory support?

YES

HFNC/NIV — Continue oxygen

Intubate if needed — Arrange descent

↓

Urgent CASEVAC

SpO_2 < 85% despite oxygen

Severe respiratory distress & cyanosis

Confusion/altered sensorium

Frothy sputum

Associated HACE suspected

Principles of Evacuation

ɜ Transport	During Transport
bilize airway rt oxygen ːp patient warm	**Continue:** • Oxygen therapy, monitoring • Upright positioning & warmth **Avoid:** • Exertion & Delays

CASEVAC Algorithm

HAPE diagnosed
↓
Assess severity
↓
Severe hypoxia/distress?

YES	NO
Urgent CASEVAC	Continue treatment
High-flow oxygen	Monitor closely
NIV/intubation if required	Plan descent

↓
Continuous monitoring during transport

Practical Pearls

ange descent promptly ɿitor SpO_2 continuously	Ignore worsening hypoxia Miss coexisting HACE

Operational Pearls

- "HAPE can occur in fit individuals."
- "Early oxygen dramatically improves survival."
- "When in doubt – descend."
- "Breathlessness with crackles at altitude is HAPE until proven otherwise."

ested reading

ʒärtsch P, Swenson ER. Acute high-altitude illnesses. N Engl J Med. 2013;368(24):2294-2302.
ʌaggiorini M. High altitude-induced pulmonary oedema. Cardiovasc Res. 2006;72(1):41-50.

CHAPTER 3 HIGH-ALTITUDE PULMONARY EDEMA (HAPE)

HAPE is a potentially fatal, non-cardiogenic pulmonary edema that develops after rapid ascent to high altitude (usually > 2500 m). Early recognition, oxygen and descent are life-saving.

RED FLAGS (Think HAPE)

- Breathlessness at rest
- SpO_2 < 85% on room air
- Tachypnea > 30/min
- Crackles in lungs
- Tachycardia > 110/min
- Pink, frothy sputum
- Cyanosis
- Severe fatigue/exhaustion
- Confusion / agitation

1. RECOGNITION

Typical Onset

2–4 days after rapid ascent (can be earlier)

Risk Factors

- Rapid ascent
- Previous HAPE
- High altitude (>2500 m)
- Oveexertion
- Cold exposure
- Male > female

Typical Features

- Breathlessness at rest
- Dry cough → may become frothy sputum
- Chest tightness
- Fatigue, weakness
- Poor exercise tolerance
- Decreased urine output
- Disturbed sleep

Key Clinical Signs

- Tachypnea, use of accessory muscles
- Fine to coarse crackles
- Tachycardia
- Hypoxemia (low SpO_2)
- Hypertension or normal BP
- Frothy pink sputum (late)
- Cyanosis
- No fever

Pathophysiology (Key Points)

- Hypoxic pulmonary vasoconstriction is exaggerated in susceptible individuals.
- ↑ Pulmonary artery pressure → stress failure of capillaries.
- Leakage of fluid into alveoli → impaired → hypoxemia.

Key Message

Think HAPE in any person with new-onset breathlessness at rest after rapid ascent, especially with crackles and low SpO_2.

2. DIFFERENTIAL DIAGNOSIS

Condition	Key Clues	Features Against HAPE
HAPE	Recent rapid ascent, exertion, nonproductive cough → frothy sputum, improves with descent, no fever	—
Pneumonia	Fever, productive cough, localized chest pain, leukocytosis	Recent rapid ascent, no fever, bilateral infiltrates, rapid response to descent
Acute Exacerbation of COPD / Asthma	History of COPD/asthma, wheeze, prolonged expiration	No past history, fine crackles, no wheeze
Pulmonary Embolism (High Altitude)	Sudden onset, pleuritic chest pain, hemoptysis, risk factors	Bilateral crackles, frothy sputum, improves with descent
Cardiogenic Pulmonary Edema	History of heart disease, orthopnea, PND, raised JVP, S3 gallop	Normal heart exam, normal JVP, no pedal edema

Useful Monitoring

- SpO_2 (continuous)
- Reart rateư
- Blood pressure
- Urine output
- Mental status

Expected Response

- Improvement within 30–60 min of oxygen + nifedipine + rest
- Falling RR, improving SpO_2
- Decrease in crackles and dyspnea

3. OXYGEN & DRUG THERAPY

A. OXYGEN THERAPY

- Start immediately
- Target SpO_2 > 90%
- Delivery options:

Device	Flow Rate
Nasal prongs	2–6 L/min
Simple face mask	6–10 L/min
Non-rebreather mask	10–15 L/min
HFNC	High flow
NIV (CPAP/BiPAP)	As needed
Intubation	If failing

Consider NIV if:

- Persistent hypoxemia
- Moderate–severe distress
- Fatigue/impending failure

B. DRUG THERAPY

1. **NIFEDIPINE (First line)**

- **Mechanism:** Pulmonary vasodilation
- **Dose:** 30 mg PO (sustained release) every 8–12 hourly
- Continue until improvement and descent
- Avoid if SBP < 100 mmHg

2. **PHOSPHODIESTERASE-5 INHIBITOR (If Nifedipine not available)**

- Sildenafil 50 mg PO every 8 hourly

3. **SUPPORTIVE THERAPY**

- **Diuretics:** Furosemide 20–40 mg IV (if severe fluid overload)
- **Morphine:** 2–4 mg IV (anxiety, severe dyspnea)
- **Hydration:** Oral/IV as tolerated
- Treat cough (avoid sedating cough syrups)

4. HAPE ALGORITHM

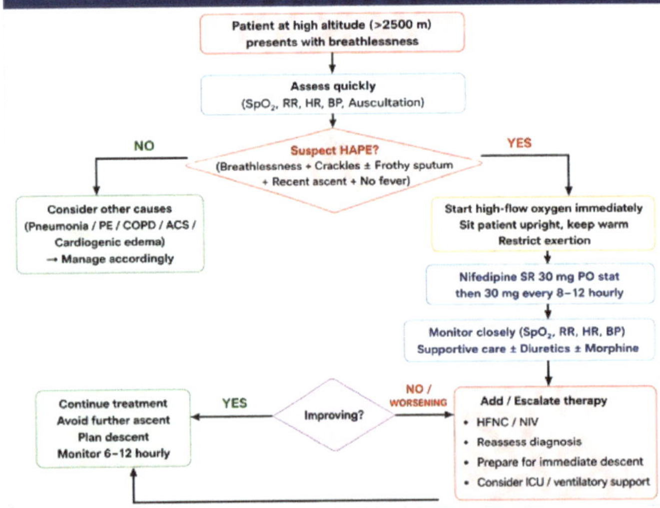

5. EVACUATION CRITERIA

IMMEDIATE DESCENT / CASEVAC IF:

- Severe breathlessness at rest
- SpO_2 < 85% despite oxygen
- Deteriorating mental status
- Hemodynamic instability
- Need for NIV / mechanical ventilation
- No improvement within 2–4 hours
- Recurrent vomiting / exhaustion
- Any sign of multi-organ dysfunction

PRINCIPLES OF EVACUATION

- Stabilize before transport (high-flow oxygen, IV access, monitoring)
- Keep patient warm (avoid hypothermia)
- Continuous monitoring during transport
- Inform receiving center early

TRANSPORT CONSIDERATIONS

- Oxygen throughout transport
- Upright / semi-recumbent position
- Avoid exertion during move
- Reassess frequently

PRACTICAL PEARLS

- HAPE can develop in anyone—fitness does not protect.
- Oxygen early, descend early.
- Nifedipine is the cornerstone drug.
- Avoid exertion and further ascent.
- When in doubt—descend.

CHAPTER 4
HIGH-ALTITUDE CEREBRAL EDEMA (HACE)

"Confusion at altitude is HACE until proven otherwise."

High-Altitude Cerebral Edema (HACE) is a life-threatening neurological emergency caused by severe altitude-related cerebral swelling. It is considered the end-stage progression of Acute Mountain Sickness (AMS).

HACE requires:

- Immediate recognition, Urgent oxygen therapy, Dexamethasone & Rapid descent/CASEVAC

Delay in treatment may rapidly lead to coma and death.

1. RECOGNITION

Definition

HACE is severe altitude illness characterized by:

- Altered mental status AND/OR ataxia occurring after recent ascent to high altitude.

Usually occurs:

- Above 3000–4000 m
- Often after untreated AMS

	!

Why HACE Occurs at High Altitude

Hypobaric hypoxia causes:

- Cerebral vasodilation & increased capillary permeability
- Cerebral edema & raised intracranial pressure
- Brain dysfunction

Risk Factors

[illegible]	[illegible]
on	Aggravates hypoxia

[illegible]
vere persistent headache
current vomiting
cal neurological deficit or seizur
creasing consciousness

Symptoms

? headache	Inability to walk	Ataxia, Confusion, Irritability
[illegible]	[illegible]	[illegible]

Important Clinical Point: "Ataxia at altitude is HACE until proven otherwise."

2. NEUROLOGICAL ASSESSMENT

Rapid Neurological Assessment

A. Mental Status: Assess: Orientation, Memory, Behaviour, Speech, Attention

B. Gait Assessment (Very Important)

Tandem Walking Test: Ask patient to Walk heel-to-toe in straight line (Abnormal gait strongly suggests HACE)

C. GCS Assessment: GCS: 15 (Mild), 13–14 (Moderate), ≤12 (Severe HACE)

D. Pupils: Check: Size, Equality, Light reaction

E. Look For Associated HAPE: Check: Breathlessness, Crackles, Severe hypoxia (HACE + HAPE commonly coexist)

Recognition Algorithm

Recent ascent >3000 m

↓

Headache / AMS symptoms

Neurolo

(Ataxia/confusion/slurred speech)

Meningitis	**Fever/neck stiffness**

YES — Suspect HACE

NO — AMS more likely

Check G

Any deterioration?

YES — Immediate treatment + descent

NO — Close monitoring

DEXAMETHASONE PROTOCOL

GOLDEN RULE: *"Oxygen + dexamethasone + descent save lives."*

Immediate Stabilization

Step 1 – Stop further ascent

Step 2 – Oxygen Therapy: *Give immediately **and target** highest achievable SpO_2*

Dexamethasone (Drug of Choice): Initial Dose: *8 mg IV/IM/PO stat THEN* **maintenance Dose** *4 mg every 6 hours*

Duration; *Continue until descent completed OR* **s***ymptoms fully resolve*

Important Notes

Improvement may occur rapidly, continue monitoring closely and descent is mandatory

Additional Measures

Position: *Head elevated*

Fluids: *Maintain hydration cautiously*

Avoid: *Sedatives, Alcohol, Exertion*

Seizure Management: Lorazepam *(4 mg IV) OR* **Midazolam** *(5–10 mg IV/IM)*

Severe HACE: *If GCS falling, Airway compromised, Respiratory failure* **then** *prepare intubation, ICU transfer* **and** *urgent CASEVAC*

HACE ALGORITHM

Patient at altitude with AMS symptoms

Neurolo

(Ataxia

YES — Suspect HACE

NO — Continue AMS treatment

↓

Check G

↓

Start oxygen immediately

↓

Give dexamethasone

8 mg stat

↓

Need airway support?

Altered sensorium

GCS < 15

Severe hypoxia

Coexisting HAPE

Inability to walk

Failure to improve rapidly

YES — Prepare intubation

NO — Monitor closely

↓

Arrange immediate descent / CASEVAC

↓

Continuous monitoring

Severe HACE Algorithm

Severe HACE suspected
(GCS falling/coma/seizures)
↓
High-flow oxygen
↓
Dexamethasone 8 mg IV stat
↓
Secure airway if needed
↓
Monitor:
GCS/SpO_2/RR/BP
↓
Urgent CASEVAC
ICU transfer

ıazolam	5–10 mg IV/IM	Seizures

EVACUATION CRITERIA

Immediate Descent / CASEVAC Required In ALL HACE Patients

Because HACE is potentially fatal.

Principles of Evacuation

CASEVAC Algorithm

HACE suspected
↓
Start oxygen + dexamethasone
↓
Assess airway + GCS
↓

YES
Urgent CASEVAC
ICU transfer
↓
Continuous monitoring during transport

NO
Arrange descent
Monitor continuously

Practic

at ataxia as HACE e oxygen immediately rt dexamethasone early and arrange rapid descen	Delay evacuation Miss coexisting HAPE Ignore behavioural changes

Operational Pearls

- "Ataxia is the hallmark of HACE & any confusion at altitude is dangerous."
- "Dexamethasone buys time – descent saves life."
- "Early treatment dramatically improves survival."

ested reading

Hackett PH, Roach RC. High-altitude cerebral edema. High Alt Med Biol. 2004;5(2):136-146.

Wilson MH, Newman S, Imray CH. The cerebral effects of ascent to high altitudes. Lancet Neurol.

CHAPTER 4: HIGH-ALTITUDE CEREBRAL EDEMA (HACE)

GOLDEN RULE: OXYGEN + DEXAMETHASONE + DESCENT = LIFE

1. RECOGNITION

Typical Onset

Usually 1–4 days after ascent above 3000–4000 m

Often follows untreated AMS

Early Symptoms

Severe headache
- Fatigue
- Nausea / vomiting
- Poor coordination
- Sleep disturbance

Key Neurological Features

Ataxia (unsteady gait)
- Confusion
- Irritability / altered behavior
- Slurred speech
- Poor concentration
- Drowsiness

Risk Factors
- Rapid ascent
- Previous HACE
- Untreated AMS
- Exertion
- Poor acclimatization
- Severe hypoxia

RED FLAG SIGNS (Think HACE)
- Ataxia (most important)
- Altered sensorium
- GCS < 15
- Severe persistent headache
- Recurrent vomiting
- Focal neurological deficit
- Seizures
- Decreasing consciousness

KEY MESSAGE: Ataxia at altitude is HACE until proven otherwise.

2. NEUROLOGICAL ASSESSMENT

A. MENTAL STATUS — Assess orientation, memory, behavior, speech, attention.

B. GAIT ASSESSMENT (Tandem Walking Test) — Ask patient to walk heel-to-toe in a straight line. Any imbalance = Abnormal.

C. GCS ASSESSMENT

15	Mild
13–14	Moderate
≤ 12	**Severe HACE**

D. PUPILS — Check size, equality and reaction to light.

E. LOOK FOR ASSOCIATED HAPE — Check for breathlessness, crackles, severe hypoxia.

IMPORTANT MONITORING

GCS (serial) • SpO_2 (continuous) • RR (hourly) • BP (hourly)
Pupils (serial) • Gait (repeat) • Urine output (4-hourly)

DIFFERENTIAL DIAGNOSIS

Condition	Key Clues	Features Against HACE
Pneumonia	Fever, productive cough, localized chest pain	Focal consolidation, fever common
Stroke	Sudden focal deficit, vascular risk factors	Usually focal signs, not preceded by AMS
Meningitis / Encephalitis	Fever, neck stiffness, photophobia	Fever present, CSF changes
Hypoglycemia	Low glucose, sweaty, confusion	Glucose low
Seizure / Post-ictal	History of seizure, post-ictal confusion	Seizure witnessed
Intoxication	Alcohol / drug history	Odor / history present
Trauma	History of injury	Signs of head trauma

3. DEXAMETHASONE PROTOCOL

IMMEDIATE STABILIZATION
1. Stop further ascent
2. Give oxygen immediately
3. Keep warm, head elevated
4. Establish IV access
5. Monitor (GCS, SpO_2, RR, BP)

DEXAMETHASONE REGIMEN

Initial Dose
8 mg IV / IM / PO STAT

Then
Maintenance Dose
4 mg every 6 hours

Continue until:
- Descent completed OR
- Symptoms fully resolve

ADDITIONAL MEASURES
- Maintain hydration cautiously
- Avoid sedatives, alcohol, and exertion
- Treat seizures if present
- Look for & treat HAPE

SEIZURE MANAGEMENT
- Lorazepam 4 mg IV

OR
- Midazolam 5–10 mg IV / IM

SEVERE HACE
- GCS falling / coma
- Airway compromised
- Respiratory failure
- → Prepare intubation
- → ICU care
- → Urgent CASEVAC

DRUG DOSES (QUICK REFERENCE)

Drug	Dose	Purpose
Dexamethasone	8 mg stat then 4 mg 6-hourly	HACE
Lorazepam	4 mg IV	Seizures
Midazolam	5–10 mg IV/IM	Seizures
Oxygen	High flow	Hypoxia

4. HACE ALGORITHM

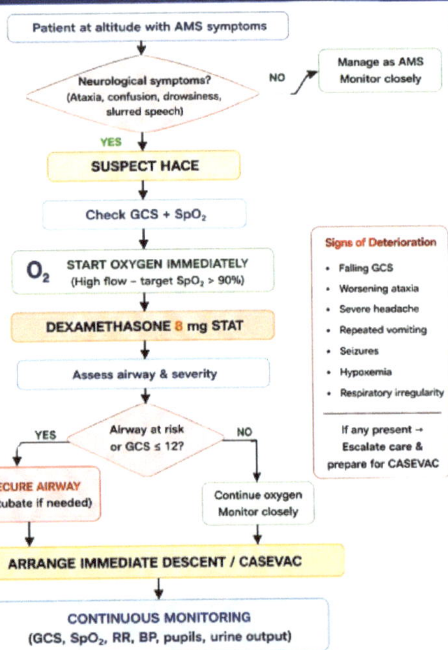

5. EVACUATION CRITERIA

IMMEDIATE DESCENT / CASEVAC IF:
- Ataxia
- Altered sensorium / confusion
- GCS < 15
- Severe hypoxia (SpO_2 < 85%)
- Seizures
- Coma / reduced consciousness
- Respiratory distress
- Coexisting HAPE
- Inability to walk
- No improvement within 1–2 hours
- Any sign of neurological deterioration

PRINCIPLES OF EVACUATION
- Stabilize before transport (oxygen, meds, IV access, monitoring)
- Keep patient warm (avoid hypothermia)
- Continue oxygen & monitoring during transport
- Head elevated (30° if possible)
- Inform receiving center early

TRANSPORT CONSIDERATIONS
- Oxygen throughout transport
- Upright / semi-recumbent position
- Avoid exertion during move
- Reassess frequently

HACE EVACUATION ALGORITHM

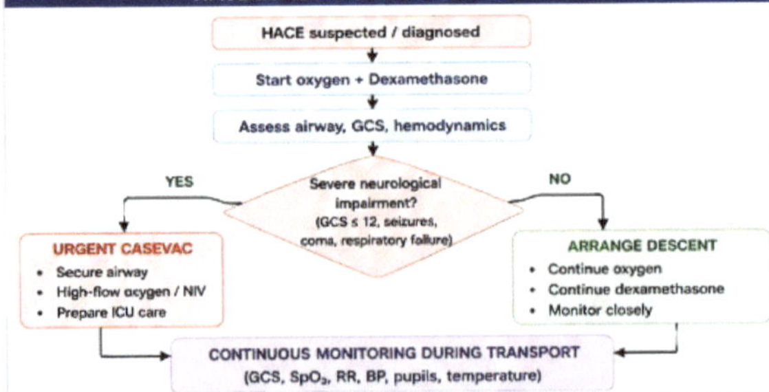

EARLY RECOGNITION • EARLY TREATMENT • EARLY DESCENT • SAVE LIVES

CHAPTER 5
BREATHLESSNESS AT HIGH ALTITUDE

"Every breathless patient at altitude is hypoxic until proven otherwise."

Breathlessness is one of the most common and potentially life-threatening presentations at high altitude. Early differentiation between High-Altitude Pulmonary Edema (HAPE), pneumonia, pulmonary embolism (PE), and cardiac causes is critical because delayed recognition rapidly increases mortality.

The priorities are:

- *Immediate oxygenation & rapid stabilization*
- *Identification of reversible causes and early referral/CASEVAC when required*

1. HAPE vs PNEUMONIA vs PE

Initial Clinical Approach

Ask:

- *Recent altitude gain?, Rate of ascent?, Fever present?*
- *Chest pain?, Haemoptysis?, Sudden onset?, Prior cardiac/lung disease?, Thrombosis risk factors?*

Common Causes of Breathlessness at High Altitude

;ondition	Key Features
[illegible]	[illegible]
ıa/COPD	Wheeze

HAPE vs Pneumonia

Crackl	**Bilateral**	**Focal/com**
[illegible]	[illegible]	[illegible]
Onset	**After ascent**	**Any time**

HAPE vs Pulmonary Embolism

[illegible]	[illegible]	[illegible]
pain	Mild	Pleuritic
[illegible]	[illegible]	[illegible]

Important Clinical Point

"Breathlessness with crackles after rapid ascent is HAPE until proven otherwise."

Rapid Evaluation

Immediate Assessment

Check: *SpO_2, Respiratory rate, Heart rate, BP, Temperature, Mental status*

Physical Examination

- ***Respiratory:*** *Crackles, wheeze, air entry, accessory muscle use*
-

Red Flag Signs

$SpO_2 < 85\%$
Severe respiratory distre
Altered sensorium
Frothy sputum
Exhaustion, RR > 30/min

Bedside Investigations

	[illegible]
	evere hypoxia

2. OXYGENATION STRATEGY

GOLDEN RULE: *"Correct hypoxia first – diagnosis can follow."*

Oxygen Therapy Principles

Start oxygen immediately in: Severe breathlessness, $SpO_2 < 90\%$, Suspected HAPE, Altered sensorium, Shock

Oxygen Targets

ıdition	Target SpO_2

Escalation of Oxygen Therapy

Hypoxia detected
↓
Nasal oxygen
↓

YES — Continue monitoring

NO — Face mask/NRBM
↓
Persistent hypoxia?
↓
HFNC/NIV
↓
Failure?
↓
Intubation

NRBM	**10–15 l**	**Severe hypoxia**

Positioning

Keep patient: Upright, Warm, Resting

Avoid: Exertion, Further ascent

3. STABILIZATION

A. Initial Stabilization

ABCDE Approach

- **Airway:** Assess: Ability to speak, Secretions, Reduced consciousness
- **Prepare airway if: GCS falling, Exhaustion, Respiratory failure**

Breathing: Immediate Actions to be taken are High-flow oxygen, Monitor SpO_2 continuously, Respiratory monitoring, Sit upright

Circulation

- **Assess:** Pulse, BP, Perfusion, Urine output
- **IV Access:** Two large-bore cannulas if unstable

Disability: Check GCS, Confusion, Seizures, Ataxia

Exposure: Assess for Hypothermia, Trauma, Frostbite

B. Disease-Specific Stabilization

- **If HAPE Suspected:** Rest, Restrict exertion, Plan descent, give oxygen and start Nifedipine
- **If Pneumonia Suspected: Give** oxygen, start antibiotics, give fluids cautiously and do fever control
- **If PE Suspected: Give** oxygen, s ... rral

Monitoring

ıeter	ıency
	l

Signs of Deterioration

Exhaustion, Increasing RR, Falling SpO_2 or Cyanosis

Hypotension and Altered sensorium

Stabilization Algorithm

Breathless patient
↓
ABCDE assessment
↓
Start o:
↓
Severe (

YES	NO
NRBM/HFNC	Face mask/nasal O_2
IV acce:	

↓
Identify
↓
Start cause-specific treatment
↓
Monitor response
↓

Severe HAPE suspected
Need for HFNC/NIV/intubation
Hemodynamic instability
Suspected PE

Severe pneumonia/sepsis
Respiratory exhaustion
No improvement within 2–4 hrs

YES	NO
Continue care	Escalate support
Plan descent	Prepare CASEVAC

Before

ize First	ng Transport
ygen ongoing & Keep patient warm	**inue:** Oxygen therapy, Monitoring, Upright
ccess secured & monitoring attached	ioning, warmth

Referral Algorithm

Breathless patient stabilized
↓

GOOD	POOR
Continue care	Need advanced support?
Plan descent	↓
Observation	YES → CASEVAC

↓
ICU/advanced respiratory care

Practical Pearls

pect HAPE after rapid ascent	erfigurate suspected HAPE
itor SpO_2 continuously	ss PE in sudden collapse& ignore altered sensorium
p patient upright & reassess frequently	lay evacuation in worsening hypoxia

Operational Pearls

- "Hypoxia kills faster at altitude."
- "Crackles + hypoxia + recent ascent = HAPE until proven otherwise."
- "Correct oxygenation before definitive diagnosis and Early referral prevents respiratory collapse."

Konstantinides SV, Meyer G, Becattini C, et al. ESC Guidelines for acute pulmonary embolism. Eur Heart J. 2020;41(4):543-603.
O'Driscoll BR, Howard LS, Earis J, Mak V. BTS guideline for oxygen use in adults. Thorax. 2017;72(Suppl 1).

CHAPTER 5: BREATHLESSNESS AT HIGH ALTITUDE

GOLDEN RULE: CORRECT HYPOXIA FIRST – DIAGNOSIS CAN FOLLOW

1. HAPE vs PNEUMONIA vs PE

INITIAL QUESTIONS

- Recent altitude gain?
- Rate of ascent?
- Fever present?
- Cough – dry or productive?
- Chest pain?
- Hemoptysis?
- Sudden onset?
- Thrombosis risk factors?
- Past cardiac / lung disease?

RED FLAG SIGNS

- $SpO_2 < 85\%$
- Severe respiratory distress
- Cyanosis
- Hypotension
- Altered sensorium
- Frothy sputum
- RR > 30/min
- Exhaustion
- Chest pain (PE/ACS)

COMPARISON TABLE

FEATURE	HAPE	PNEUMONIA	PE
Onset	Hours–Days after ascent	Any time	Sudden
Fever	Usually absent	Common	Usually absent
Cough	Dry / frothy	Productive	Dry / may have hemoptysis
Chest Pain	Mild / tightness	Pleuritic (may occur)	Pleuritic (common)
Crackles	Bilateral, basal	Focal / lobar common	None / rare
Hemoptysis	Rare	Uncommon	May occur
DVT Risk Factors	Absent	Absent	Often present
Response to Oxygen	Rapid	Partial	Variable
Response to Descent	Rapid	Slow	No change

RAPID EVALUATION

Check: SpO_2 • RR • HR BP • Temperature • Mental status

Examine: Chest (crackles/wheeze) • Heart (JVP, HS) • Extremities

BEDSIDE INVESTIGATIONS

- Pulse oximetry (continuous)
- ECG – look for arrhythmia / right heart strain / ischemia
- Chest X-ray – infiltrates / edema
- ABG (if severe hypoxia)
- Lung / cardiac ultrasound (if available)
- Blood tests as available

2. OXYGENATION STRATEGY

OXYGEN TARGETS

- General patients: $SpO_2 > 90\%$
- Severe hypoxia: Highest achievable
- COPD risk: SpO_2 88–92%

OXYGEN DELIVERY DEVICES

DEVICE	FLOW RATE	INDICATION
Nasal prongs	2–6 L/min	Mild hypoxia
Simple face mask	6–10 L/min	Moderate distress
Non-rebreather mask (NRBM)	10–15 L/min	Severe hypoxia
HFNC (High Flow Nasal Cannula)	High flow (30–60 L/min)	Persistent hypoxia
NIV (CPAP / BiPAP)	Variable	HAPE / resp. failure
Intubation	–	Impending collapse / resp. failure

OXYGEN ESCALATION ALGORITHM

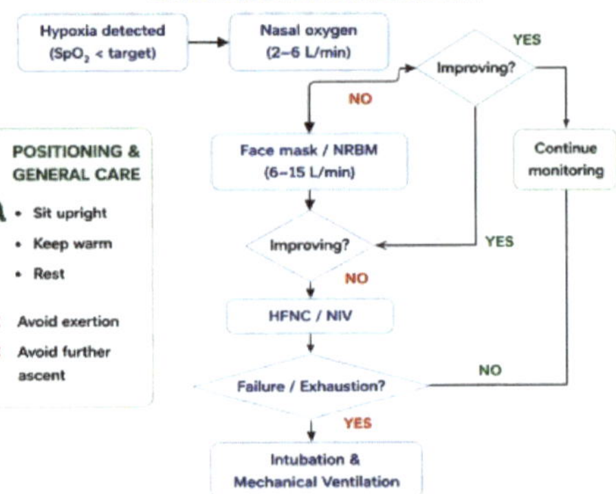

POSITIONING & GENERAL CARE

- Sit upright
- Keep warm
- Rest

× Avoid exertion

× Avoid further ascent

3. STABILIZATION

A. ABCDE APPROACH

A – Airway: Assess ability to speak, secretions, GCS. Prepare airway if GCS falling, exhaustion, or resp. failure.

B – Breathing: High-flow oxygen, monitor SpO_2, RR, work of breathing. Sit patient upright.

C – Circulation: Check pulse, BP, perfusion, capillary refill, JVP. Treat shock if present.

D – Disability: Check GCS, pupils, blood glucose. Look for confusion, seizures, ataxia (HACE).

E – Exposure: Look for hypothermia, trauma, rash, DVT signs.

B. DISEASE-SPECIFIC STABILIZATION

If HAPE suspected

- High-flow oxygen
- Nifedipine (SR 30 mg PO 12 hourly)
- Restrict exertion
- Warmth & rest
- Arrange descent

If Pneumonia suspected

- Oxygen
- Antibiotics (as per protocol)
- Fluids cautiously
- Fever control

If PE suspected

- Oxygen
- Anticoagulation (if no contraindication)
- Urgent imaging / specialist referral
- Analgesia for pain

MONITORING

- SpO_2 – Continuous
- HR – Hourly
- HR – Hourly
- BP – Hourly
- GCS – Serial

SIGNS OF DETERIORATION

- Falling SpO_2
- Increasing RR
- Exhaustion
- Hypotension
- Altered sensorium
- Cyanosis
- Arrhythmia
- Poor urine output
- No improvement

4. REFERRAL CRITERIA

IMMEDIATE REFERRAL / CASEVAC IF:

- $SpO_2 < 85\%$ despite oxygen
- Severe HAPE suspected
- Need for HFNC / NIV / Intubation
- Hemodynamic instability
- Suspected PE
- Altered sensorium / HACE
- Coexisting HAPE + HACE
- Severe pneumonia / sepsis
- Respiratory exhaustion
- No improvement within 2–4 hours

BEFORE REFERRAL – STABILIZE FIRST

- High-flow oxygen
- IV access (2 large bore)
- Continuous monitoring
- Keep warm
- Essential drugs given
- Inform receiving center

DURING TRANSPORT

- Continue oxygen therapy
- Continuous monitoring
- Keep patient upright
- Keep warm & covered
- Avoid delays & exertion

TRANSPORT CONSIDERATIONS

- Oxygen throughout transport
- Upright / semi-recumbent position
- Secure all lines & monitors
- Sedate only if necessary
- Reassess frequently
- Prepare for deterioration

5. OVERALL MANAGEMENT ALGORITHM FOR BREATHLESSNESS AT HIGH ALTITUDE

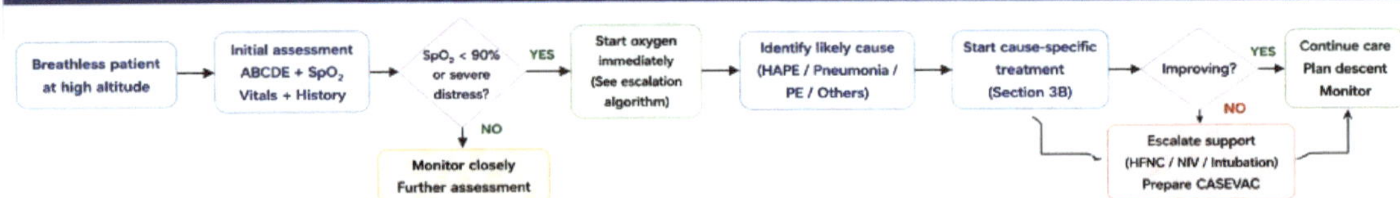

KEY PROTOCOLS (QUICK REFERENCE)

OXYGEN PROTOCOL

- Start early
- Target $SpO_2 > 90\%$
- Escalate device as needed
- Monitor continuously

HAPE PROTOCOL

- Oxygen
- Nifedipine SR 30 mg PO 12 hourly
- Rest + warmth
- Descent

PNEUMONIA PROTOCOL

- Oxygen
- Antibiotics
- Fluids cautiously
- Fever control

PE PROTOCOL

- Oxygen
- Anticoagulation (if indicated)
- Analgesia
- Urgent referral

GENERAL PROTOCOL

- ABCDE
- Monitor vitals
- Reassess frequently
- Early referral saves lives

EARLY OXYGEN • EARLY RECOGNITION • EARLY STABILIZATION • EARLY REFERRAL • SAVE LIVES

CHAPTER 6
CHEST PAIN & CARDIAC EMERGENCIES

"Chest pain at altitude is cardiac until proven otherwise."

Cardiac emergencies at high altitude may deteriorate rapidly because hypoxia increases myocardial oxygen demand, sympathetic activation, pulmonary artery pressure, and arrhythmogenic risk.

The priorities are:

- *Rapid recognition of ACS/STEMI*
- *Immediate oxygenation*
- *Early ECG acquisition*
- *Stabilization of arrhythmias/shock*
- *Timely reperfusion and evacuation*

1. ACS AT ALTITUDE

Why ACS Worsens at High Altitude

Hypobaric hypoxia causes:

- *Increased heart rate, Increased myocardial oxygen demand, Increased sympathetic activity, Vasoconstriction*
- *Polycythaemia and thrombosis risk*

These factors may:

- *Trigger plaque rupture, worsen ischemia, Increase arrhythmias, Precipitate heart failure/shock*

Common Presentations

[illegible]	[illegible]
›genic shock	Hypotension + hypoperfusion

athlessness ısea/vomiting ɒitations, Syncope	Pulmonary edema, Altered sensorium, Shock Arrhythmias, ST elevation	► AF with instability Wide complex tachycardia Bradycardia with shock

Initial Evaluation

Immediate Steps

ABCDE assessment, oxygen if hypoxic, IV access, 12-lead ECG within 30 minutes, Blood glucose, Cardiac monitoring

Important Clinical Point: "Do not dismiss chest pain as altitude-related fatigue."

2. ECG CHANGES

Common ECG Changes at High Altitude

[illegible]	[illegible]
:hanges	Hypoxia/ischemia

STEMI Recognition

STEMI Criteria

ST elevation in ≥2 contiguous leads OR **New LBBB with ischemic symptoms**

sed JVP, Clear lungs	ST depression V1–V3 Tall R waves posteriorly

ECG Monitoring

Continuous monitoring in:

- ACS
- Arrhythmias
- Shock
- Severe hypoxia

3. STEMI PROTOCOL

GOLDEN RULE: "Time is myocardium."

Immediate STEMI Management

A. Oxygen: Give only if: SpO_2 < 90%, breathlessness, shock

B. Aspirin : Dose– 325 mg chewed stat

C. Second Antiplatelet: Clopidogrel– 300–600 mg loading OR **Ticagrelor–** 180 mg loading

D. Anticoagulation: Enoxaparin: As per STEMI protocol

E. Nitrates: GTN, only if BP is stable **and** no RV infarction (Avoid if there is hypotension, RV MI, severe aortic stenosis)

F. Thrombolysis: If PCI unavailable within recommended timelines.

Common Thrombolytics

bolysis Contraindications ive bleeding ent stroke or intracranial bleed	**st-Thrombolysis Monitoring** nitor: • ECG resolution

STEMI Algorithm

Chest pain patient
↓
12-lead
↓
ST elev

YES NO
STEMI protocol | Evaluate NSTEMI/ other causes
↓
Aspirin + antiplatelet
Oxygen if hypoxic
Anticoagulation
↓

YES NO
Transfer for PCI | Thrombolysis
↓
Monitor continuously
Prepare evacuation

4. ARRHYTHMIAS

Common Arrhythmias at Altitude

	Hypoxia/stress

Initial Approach

Assess Stability: *Signs of instability: Hypotension, Shock, Chest pain, Altered sensorium, Severe hypoxia*

Stable SVT: Vagal manoeuvres *THEN* ***Adenosine–*** *6 mg rapid IV then 12 mg if required*

Unstable SVT: Immediate synchronized cardioversion

VT/VF: Initiation of Immediate treatment as per ACLS protocol

Shockable rhythm: *Defibrillation, CPR, Adrenaline, Amiodarone*

AF Management

- ***Stable:*** *Rate control, Oxygen, Treat underlying hypoxia*
- ***Unstable:*** *Cardioversion*

Arrhythmia Algorithm

Arrhythmia detected
↓
Assess stability
↓
Unstable?

YES — *Cardioversion/ ACLS*
↓
Correct hypoxia
Monitor continuously
Prepare referral if needed

NO — *ECG analysis* — *Treat rhythm*

Adrena	***1 mg IV***	***iac arrest***

5. CARDIOGENIC SHOCK

Definition: *Cardiogenic shock is inadequate tissue perfusion due to severe cardiac dysfunction*

Clinical

Hypotension, Cold extremities, Pulmonary edema, Altered sensorium, Oliguria, Tachycardia

Common Causes at Altitude

thmias	*'requent*

Immediate Management

A. Oxygen: *High-flow oxygen*

B. Monitoring: *ECG, BP, Urine output, SpO_2*

C. Vasopressors/Inotropes

- ***Noradrenaline:*** *Preferred vasopressor*
- ***Dobutamine:*** *If poor cardiac output*

D. Avoid Excess Fluids

Especially in Pulmonary edema & LV dysfunction

E. Urgent Reperfusion/Transfer

Cardiogenic Shock Algorithm

Hypotension + chest pain

Signs o
(cold ex
↓
Suspect cardiogenic shock
↓
High-flow oxygen
Continu
IV acces

ECG + STEMI evaluation
↓
Start vasopressor support
Avoid fluid overload
↓
Urgent ICU referral / CASEVAC

STEMI
Cardiogenic shock
Sustained arrhythmia
VT/VF

Recurrent chest pain
Failed thrombolysis
Hemodynamic instability

Practical Pearls

at hypoxia aggressively ognize STEMI rapidly nitor continuously ange early evacuation	Ignore arrhythmias Overhydrate pulmonary edema patients Miss RV infarction Delay cardioversion in unstable patients

Operational Pearls

- "Hypoxia increases arrhythmia risk."
- "Time lost is myocardium lost."
- "Early ECG saves lives."
- "Cardiogenic shock at altitude deteriorates rapidly."

banez B, James S, Agewall S, et al. ESC Guidelines for STEMI management. Eur Heart J. 2018;39(2):119-177.
'anchal AR, Bartos JA, Cabanas JG, et al. 2020 AHA Guidelines for CPR and ECC. Circulation.
2020;142(16_suppl_2): S366-S468.

CHAPTER 6: CHEST PAIN & CARDIAC EMERGENCIES

GOLDEN RULE: CHEST PAIN AT ALTITUDE IS CARDIAC UNTIL PROVEN OTHERWISE.

1. ACS AT ALTITUDE

Why ACS Worsens at High Altitude

- ↑ Heart rate & myocardial oxygen demand
- Hypoxia, vasoconstriction
- Polycythemia & thrombosis risk
- ↑ Sympathetic activity
- Triggers plaque rupture, ischemia, arrhythmias, heart failure/shock

Typical Symptoms

- Central chest pain / pressure
- Radiation to arm / jaw / back
- Sweating
- Breathlessness
- Nausea / vomiting
- Palpitations
- Syncope

Presentations

- STEMI – ST elevation
- NSTEMI – Troponin rise
- Unstable angina – No biomarker rise
- Cardiogenic shock – Hypotension, poor perfusion

High-Risk Features

- Hypotension
- Severe hypoxia
- Arrhythmias
- Pulmonary edema
- Altered sensorium
- Ongoing chest pain
- ST elevation
- Shock
- Exhaustion

Initial Evaluation – Do Immediately

ABCDE assessment · Oxygen if SpO_2 < 90% · IV access · 12-lead ECG within 10 min · Cardiac monitoring · Check blood glucose

IMPORTANT POINT: Do not dismiss chest pain as altitude-related fatigue.

2. ECG CHANGES

Common ECG Changes at High Altitude

- Sinus tachycardia
- Right axis deviation
- T-wave inversion (RV strain)
- ST-T changes (hypoxia/ischemia)
- Premature beats

Dangerous ECG Findings

- ST elevation
- Sustained VT / VF
- Complete heart block
- AF with instability
- Wide complex tachycardia
- Bradycardia with shock

STEMI Recognition

ST elevation in ≥2 contiguous leads
OR
New LBBB with ischemic symptoms

RV Infarction Clues

- Inferior STEMI
- Hypotension
- Raised JVP
- Clear lungs

Posterior MI Clues

- ST depression V1–V3
- Tall R waves in V1–V3

ECG Monitoring

Continuous monitoring in ACS, arrhythmias, shock, severe hypoxia.

3. STEMI PROTOCOL

A OXYGEN (Give only if)
- SpO_2 < 90% • Breathlessness • Shock

B ASPIRIN
- 325 mg chewed STAT

C SECOND ANTIPLATELET (Choose one)
- Clopidogrel 300–600 mg loading OR
- Ticagrelor 180 mg loading

D ANTICOAGULATION
- Enoxaparin as per STEMI protocol

E NITRATES (GTN)
- 0.4 mg SL – repeat q5 min (Max 3 doses)
- Use only if BP stable, not in RV MI
- Avoid if: Hypotension • RV infarction • Severe AS

F REPERFUSION STRATEGY

PCI AVAILABLE (Minimal delay): Transfer for Primary PCI

PCI NOT AVAILABLE (Delay >120 min): Thrombolysis

Common Thrombolytics

Drug	Dose
Tenecteplase	Weight-based single IV bolus
Streptokinase	1.5 million IU IV over 60 min

Thrombolysis Contraindications

- Active internal bleeding
- Recent stroke / ICH
- Intracranial pathology
- Severe uncontrolled HTN
- Known bleeding disorder

After Thrombolysis – Monitor

ECG resolution · Arrhythmias · Shock · Reperfusion pain · Bleeding

STEMI ALGORITHM

Chest pain patient
↓
12-lead ECG
↓
ST elevation?

- YES → STEMI Protocol → Aspirin + Antiplatelet / Oxygen if hypoxic / Anticoagulation / Monitor continuously → PCI available rapidly?
  - YES → Transfer for Primary PCI
  - NO → Give Thrombolysis
  - → Monitor continuously / Prepare evacuation / referral
- NO → Evaluate NSTEMI / Unstable Angina / Other causes → Treat accordingly / Monitor closely

4. ARRHYTHMIAS

Common Arrhythmias at Altitude

- Sinus tachycardia (most common)
- Supraventricular tachycardia (SVT)
- Atrial fibrillation (AF)
- Ventricular tachycardia (VT)
- Ventricular fibrillation (VF)
- Bradycardia / Heart block

Initial Approach

1. Assess Stability

Hypotension · Shock · Chest pain · Altered sensorium · Severe hypoxia

UNSTABLE (Any one present) → Immediate Synchronized Cardioversion → Follow ACLS if needed

STABLE → 2. Identify Rhythm

- **SVT (Regular Narrow QRS)**
  - Vagal maneuvers
  - Adenosine 6 mg IV rapid bolus
  - If no response: Adenosine 12 mg IV
- **AF**
  - Rate control (e.g., Beta blocker / Diltiazem)
  - Oxygen
  - Treat underlying cause
  - If unstable → Cardioversion
- **VT / VF**
  - Follow ACLS protocol
  - Shockable rhythm → Defibrillate
  - Amiodarone 300 mg IV
- **Bradycardia**
  - Atropine 0.6 mg IV
  - Repeat q3–5 min (max 3 mg)
  - If ineffective → Pacing

3. Correct Hypoxia & Electrolytes
4. Monitor Continuously
5. Prepare Referral if Needed

Drug Box (Quick Reference)

Drug	Dose	Use
Adenosine	6 mg → 12 mg IV	SVT
Amiodarone	300 mg IV bolus	VT/VF
Adrenaline	1 mg IV q3–5 min	Cardiac arrest
GTN	0.4 mg SL	ACS (if BP stable)
Aspirin	325 mg chewed	STEMI
Atropine	0.6 mg IV	Bradycardia

ACLS Pearls at Altitude

- Hypoxia worsens arrhythmias – correct early.
- High-quality CPR, minimal interruptions.
- Defbirillate early for VT/VF.
- Treat reversible causes (H's & T's).

5. CARDIOGENIC SHOCK

Definition

Inadequate tissue perfusion due to severe cardiac dysfunction.

Clinical Features

- Hypotension (SBP < 90 mmHg)
- Cold clammy extremities
- Pulmonary edema
- Altered sensorium
- Oligurio (< 0.5 mL/kg/h)
- Tachycardia / weak pulse

Common Causes

- STEMI (most common)
- Arrhythmias
- Right ventricular infarction
- Severe hypoxia
- Acute heart failure

Immediate Management

A Oxygen – High-flow
B Monitoring – ECG, BP, SpO_2, Urine output
C IV Access – Two large bore cannulas
D Vasopressors / Inotropes
- Noradrenaline (preferred)
- Dobutamine (if low output)

E Avoid Excess Fluids (pulmonary edema)
F Treat Cause – Reperfusion / Rhythm control

Targets

- MAP ≥ 65 mmHg
- SpO_2 > 90%
- Urine output > 0.5 mL/kg/h
- Warm peripheries
- Improving sensorium

↓

Urgent Reperfusion / Transfer to Higher Center

OVERALL MANAGEMENT ALGORITHM FOR CHEST PAIN & CARDIAC EMERGENCIES

Patient with Chest Pain / Palpitations / Collapse at High Altitude
↓
ABCDE Assessment
Check: SpO_2, BP, HR, RR, GCS • Give Oxygen if SpO_2 < 90% • IV Access • Monitor
12-lead ECG within 10 minutes

- **STEMI**: Go to STEMI Protocol
- **NSTEMI / Unstable Angina**: Antiplatelet, Anticoagulation, Pain relief, Monitor, Refer
- **Arrhythmia**: Assess Stability, Treat per Arrhythmia Algorithm
- **Cardiogenic Shock**: Start Shock Management Algorithm
- **Other Causes**: Evaluate: Pneumonia, PE, HAPE, GI / MSK etc.

↓
Monitor Response

- Stable / Improving → Continue Treatment / Plan Descent / Monitor Closely
- Unstable / Not Improving → Escalate Support / Prepare CASEVAC / Refer to Higher Center

REFERRAL CRITERIA (CASEVAC REQUIRED IF)

- STEMI
- Cardiogenic shock
- Sustained arrhythmia (VT / VF / unstable SVT)
- Severe hypoxia (SpO_2 < 85% despite O_2)
- Pulmonary edema
- Hemodynamic instability
- Recurrent / ongoing chest pain
- Failed thrombolysis
- Need for PCI / ICU care
- Altered sensorium
- High-risk PE suspected

Before Referral

- ✓ Oxygen ongoing
- ✓ IV access secured
- ✓ Monitoring attached
- ✓ Essential drugs given
- ✓ Inform receiving center

EARLY ECG • EARLY OXYGEN • EARLY TREATMENT • EARLY REFERRAL • SAVE MYOCARDIUM, SAVE LIVES

CHAPTER 7
STROKE, SEIZURES & ALTERED SENSORIUM

"Any altered sensorium at altitude is a neurological emergency until proven otherwise."

Neurological emergencies at high altitude may result from:

- *Hypoxia, Cerebral edema, Thrombosis, Stroke, Seizures, Metabolic disturbances*

Delayed recognition rapidly increases morbidity and mortality.
The priorities are:

- *Rapid neurological assessment*
- *Airway protection*
- *Correction of hypoxia*
- *Identification of reversible causes and early evacuation*

FAST Assessment

GCS decline
Severe headache
Seizures

Altered behaviour

1. STROKE RECOGNITION

Why Stroke Risk Increases at High Altitude

Hypoxic

-
- *Polycythaemia, Endothelial dysfunction*
- *Cerebral blood flow abnormalities*

These increase the risk of:

-
-
- *Haemorrhagic stroke*

Common Stroke Presentations

deviation	*Stroke clue*

Important Clinical Point: *"Stroke and HACE may coexist at altitude."*

Immediate Evaluation

Check: *GCS, Pupils, Limb power, Speech, Blood glucose, SpO_2*
Initial Imaging: *Preferred initial imaging is CT brain but best is MRI brain, if available and if time permits*

Stroke Recognition Algorithm

Neurological symptoms
↓

YES — *Suspect stroke*
↓
Check: GCS/SpO_2/glucose
↓
Stabilize ABCDE
↓
Urgent neuroimaging
↓
Ischemic vs haemorrhagic stroke

NO — *Evaluate other causes*

	35 mg IV bolus

CHEMIC STROKE ONLY (IF NO
AINDICATIONS FOR) THROMBOLYSIS

Ischemic Stroke	
rnative mbolysis	Alteplase 0.9 mg/kg IV (max 90 mg)
rnative BP rol	Nicardipine infusion 5 mg/hr IV

Haemorrhagic Stroke	
Raised ICP	nitol 20%: 0.5–1 g/kg
Warfarin reversal	min K 10 mg IV + PCC

2. CVT SUSPICION

Why CVT is Important at Altitude

High altitude predisposes to:

- **Dehydration, Polycythaemia, Hyper viscosity, Venous thrombosis**

Clinical Features Suggestive of CVT

Severe headache

New-onset seizures, Papilledema

Focal deficits, Altered sensorium, Recurrent vomiting

Preferred Imaging: CT Venography OR **MR Venography**

g patient	pical

Immediate Management

Oxygen, hydration cautiously, anticoagulation if confirmed, seizure control, ICU referral if severe

Important Clinical Point: "New headache with seizures at altitude should raise suspicion for CVST."

CVT Suspicion Algorithm

Headache + neurological symptoms

Seizure

YES → Suspect CVST → CT/MR → Confirm

NO → Evaluate other causes

YES → Start anticoagulation + seizure control

NO → Reassess diagnosis

Initial anticoagulation	noxaparin 1 mg/kg SC BD
Alternative ICP agent	% Hypertonic saline: 100–150 mL olus

3. SEIZURE PROTOCOL

Initial Seizure Management

Immediate Priorities

Protect airway, Prevent injury, Give oxygen, Check glucose, Monitor vitals

First-Line Therapy: Lorazepam – 4 mg IV slow OR **Midazolam**– 5–10 mg IM/IV

Persistent Seizure: Levetiracetam– 20–60 mg/kg IV OR **Valproate**– 20–40 mg/kg IV

Seizure Protocol Algorithm

Seizure detected
↓
Protect airway
Give oxygen
Check g
↓
Seizure ongoing?

YES NO
Lorazepam 4 mg IV Monitor closely
OR Mid
↓

YES NO
Levetiracetam/ Observation
Valproate Treat cause
↓
Status epilepticus?
↓
ICU referral

Hypoglycaemia	Revers
Electrolyte imb	Commo

mportant Monitoring

4. STATUS EPILEPTICUS

Definition

Continuous seizure activity lasting > 5 minutes OR recurrent seizures without recovery or gain in consciousness

Immediate Management

A. Airway & Oxygen: Give High-flow oxygen **& perform** suction if needed

B. Benzodiazepines: Lorazepam- 4 mg IV (may repeat once)

C. Second-Line Drugs: Levetiracetam- 20–60 mg/kg IV OR **Valproate-** 20–40 mg/kg IV OR **Phenytoin-** 20 mg/kg IV

Refractory Status: Prepare for Intubation, ICU transfer **and** sedation infusion

Status

Seizure
↓
Status epilepticus
↓
Airway + oxygen + glucose check
↓
Lorazep
↓
Persistent seizure?

YES NO
Second-line AED Monitor
(Leveti
Valproa
↓
Refractory?
↓
Intubation + ICU
Urgent CASEVAC

ersistent seizure
yanosis
espiratory depression

espiratory failure
evere HACE/stroke
ability to maintain airway

5. AIRWAY PROTECTION

GOLDEN RULE: "Hypoxia and airway loss kill neurological patients early."

Airway Assessment

Assess: GCS, secretions, protective reflexes, respiratory effort

Immediate Measures

Jaw thrust/chin lift, suction secretions, oxygen, OPA/NPA if needed

Intubation Indications
Intubate if:

- Airway unprotected
- Hypoxia worsening
- Seizures recurrent
- Respiratory exhaustion

Airway Protection Algorithm

Neurological emergency
↓
Assess airway + GCS
↓

BP	Continuous

YES NO
Oxygen + monitor Suction/airway adjuncts
↓ ↓

YES NO
Prepare intubation Continue monitoring
↓
Secure airway
Arrange ICU/CASEVAC

Referra
Immedi

Stroke suspected
CVT suspected
Persistent altered sensorium
Stat
Need
Severe hypoxia
Focal neurological deficit
Recurrent seizures
Coexisting HACE

Practical Pearls

tect airway aggressively	Delay evacuation in deteriorating patients

Operational Pearls

- "Any new seizure at altitude requires urgent evaluation."
- "CVST is more common at altitude than expected."
- "Airway protection saves lives in neurological emergencies."
- "Hypoxia worsens every neurological condition."

ested reading

owers WJ, Rabinstein AA, Ackerson T, et al. Guidelines for early management of acute ischemic stroke. troke. 2019;50(12):e344–e418.
erro JM, Canhão P. Cerebral venous sinus thrombosis. Lancet Neurol. 2016;15(2):162–170.

CHAPTER 7: STROKE, SEIZURES & ALTERED SENSORIUM

GOLDEN RULE: ANY ALTERED SENSORIUM AT ALTITUDE IS A NEUROLOGICAL EMERGENCY UNTIL PROVEN OTHERWISE.

1. STROKE RECOGNITION

Why Stroke Risk Increases at High Altitude
- Hypoxemia
- Polycythemia
- Hypercoagulability
- Endothelial dysfunction
- Abnormal cerebral blood flow

Common Stroke Presentations
- Sudden weakness or numbness
- Facial deviation
- Speech difficulty
- Sudden severe headache
- Visual symptoms

FAST Assessment
- F – Facial droop
- A – Arm weakness
- S – Speech difficulty
- T – Time critical

Red Flag Signs
- Sudden focal weakness
- Aphasia / slurred speech
- GCS decline
- Severe headache
- Seizures
- Recurrent vomiting
- Unequal pupils
- Altered behavior

Immediate Evaluation
Check:
- GCS
- Pupils
- Limb power
- Speech
- Blood glucose
- SpO_2, BP, Pulse, RR

Initial Imaging (Preferred)
- CT Brain (preferred)
- MRI Brain (if available)

IMPORTANT POINT: Stroke and HACE may coexist at altitude.

STROKE RECOGNITION ALGORITHM

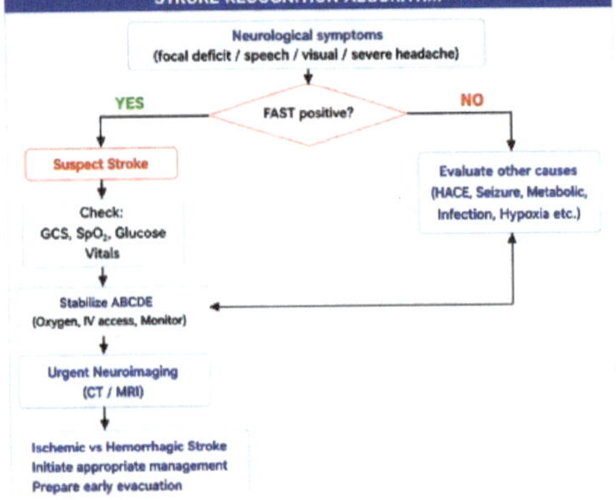

2. CVT SUSPICION

Why CVT is Important at Altitude
- Dehydration
- Polycythemia
- Hyperviscosity
- Venous thrombosis

Clinical Features Suggestive of CVT
- Severe headache
- New-onset seizures
- Papilledema
- Focal neurological deficit
- Altered sensorium
- Recurrent vomiting

Important Clues
- Severe headache – very common
- Seizures – common
- Young patient
- Recent ascent
- Raised ICP signs

Preferred Imaging
CT Venography
OR
MR Venography

Immediate Management
- ✓ Oxygen
- ✓ Hydration cautiously
- ✓ Anticoagulation (if confirmed)
- ✓ Seizure control
- ✓ ICU referral if severe

CVT SUSPICION ALGORITHM

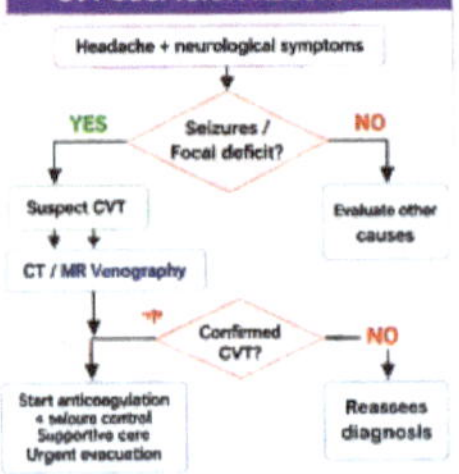

3. SEIZURE PROTOCOL

Causes of Seizures at High Altitude
HACE | Stroke/CVT | Hypoxia | Hypoglycemia | Electrolyte imbalance | CNS infection

Initial Seizure Management (First 5 Minutes)
- ✓ Protect airway
- ✓ Prevent injury
- ✓ Give oxygen (high flow)
- ✓ Check blood glucose
- ✓ Monitor vitals (SpO_2, BP, HR, RR)

First-Line Therapy
Lorazepam 4 mg IV slow
OR
Midazolam 5–10 mg IV/IM

If Seizure Persists
- Levetiracetam 20–60 mg/kg IV
OR
- Valproate 20–40 mg/kg IV

Important Monitoring
- SpO_2
- GCS
- RR
- BP
- Temperature
- Urine output

SEIZURE PROTOCOL ALGORITHM

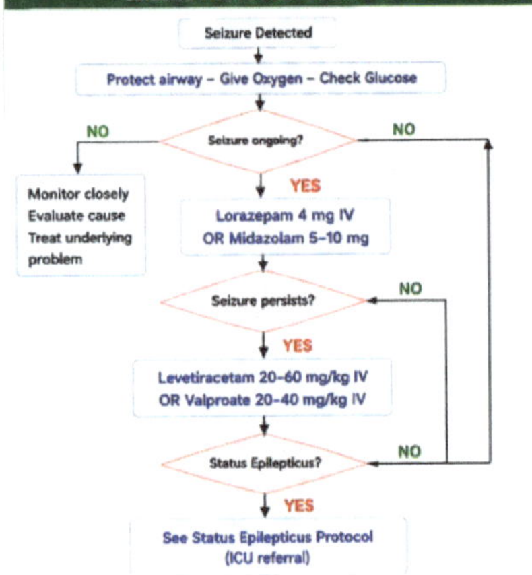

4. STATUS EPILEPTICUS

Definition
Continuous seizure activity > 5 minutes OR recurrent seizures without regaining consciousnens between them.

Red Flag Signs
- ✗ Persistent seizure
- ✗ Cyanosis
- ✗ Respiratory depression
- ✗ GCS decline
- ✗ Hypotension

1. **Airway & Oxygen – Management**
   High-flow oxygen, suction if needed
2. **Benzodiazepines (First Line)**
   Lorazepam 4 mg IV (may repeat once)
3. **Second-Line Drugs**
   - Levetiracetam 20–60 mg/kg IV OR
   - Valproate 20–40 mg/kg IV
4. **Refractory Status**
   - Prepare intubation
   - Sedation (Midazolam/Ketamine / Propofol)
   - ICU transfer – Urgent evacuation

STATUS EPILEPTICUS ALGORITHM

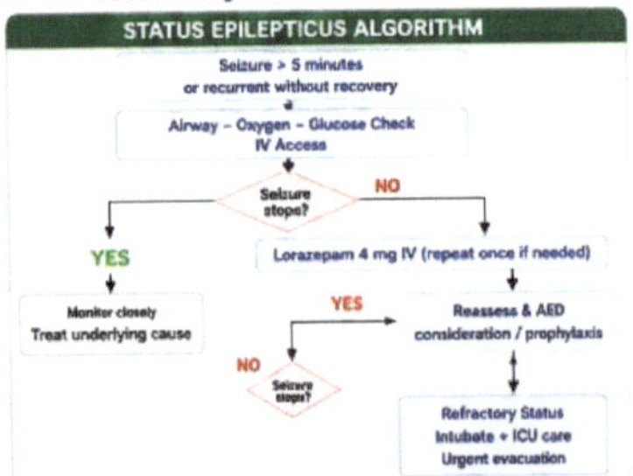

5. AIRWAY PROTECTION

Airway Assessment
- GCS
- Secretions
- Protective reflexes
- Respiratory effort

Indications for Airway Protection
- GCS ≤ 8
- Recurrent / prolonged seizures
- Aspiration risk
- Respiratory failure / hypoxia
- Severe HACE / Stroke
- Inability to maintain airway

Immediate Measures
Airway tilt–chin lift | Suction secretions | Give oxygen | OPA / NPA if needed

Intubation Indications
- Airway not protected
- Worsening hypoxia
- Refractory exhaustion
- GCS deteriorating

Monitoring After Airway Intervention
SpO_2 (Continuous) | $ETCO_2$ (if available) | BP (MAP ≥ 65 mmHg) | GCS (Serial)

AIRWAY PROTECTION ALGORITHM

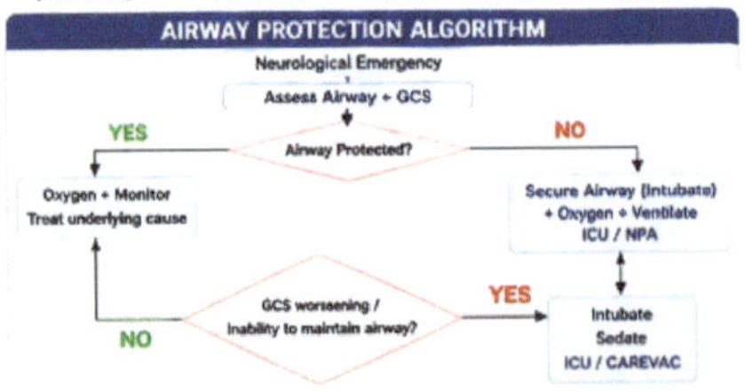

IMMEDIATE REFERRAL / CASEVAC CRITERIA

- ✓ Stroke suspected
- ✓ CVT suspected
- ✓ Persistent altered sensorium
- ✓ Status epilepticus
- ✓ Need for intubation
- ✓ Severe hypoxia
- ✓ Focal neurological deficit
- ✓ Recurrent seizures
- ✓ Coexisting HACE / HAPE
- ✓ Deteriorating GCS

PRACTICAL PEARLS

- ✓ Correct hypoxia early
- ✓ Check glucose immediately
- ✓ Monitor GCS serially
- ✓ Suspect CVT in severe headache with seizures
- ✓ Protect airway aggressively
- ✓ Early evacuation saves lives

DON'T FORGET

- ✗ Delay benzodiazepines in seizures
- ✗ Miss hypoglycemia
- ✗ Ignore subtle focal deficits
- ✗ Delay neuroimaging/referral
- ✗ Delay evacuation in deterioration

EARLY RECOGNITION | EARLY TREATMENT | AIRWAY PROTECTION | O_2 OXYGENATION | EARLY EVACUATION | SAVE LIVES

CHAPTER 8
SYNCOPE, SHOCK & COLLAPSE

"Collapse at altitude is shock until proven otherwise."
Syncope, circulatory collapse, and shock are high-risk emergencies at altitude because hypoxia rapidly worsens tissue perfusion and organ dysfunction.

The pri

-
- *Identification of shock type & correction of hypoxia*
- *Hemodynamic support & early evacuation if unstable*

Ches
Palpi
Hypo
Syncope during exertion
Severe hypoxia
Pulmonary edema

1. CARD
Why Ca

Hypoxia causes:

- *Increased sympathetic activation, tachycardia, Pulmonary hypertension,*
- *Increased myocardial oxygen demand and arrhythmogenic stress*

These may precipitate:

- *Arrhythmias, ACS/STEMI, Cardiogenic shock, Syncope, Sudden cardiac death*

Common Cardiac Causes of Collapse

genic shock	*Cold extremities/pulmonary edema*

Immediate Cardiac Assessment
Check:

- *ECG, Pulse, BP, SpO_2, Capillary refill, Mental status*

Import

Initial Cardiac Stabilization
Oxygen, ECG monitoring, IV access, Treat arrhythmias, STEMI protocol if indicated

Cardiac Collapse Algorithm
Syncope/collapse
↓
Check pulse + BP + ECG
↓

YES ***NO***
ACS/Arrhythmia/PE *Evaluate other causes*
↓
Stabilize ABCDE
Oxygen + monitoring
↓
Shock present?
↓
Start shock management
Prepare referral

2. SEPTIC SHOCK

UTI	Dysuria/fever

Why Sepsis is Dangerous at Altitude

Hypoxia worsens:

- *Tissue oxygen delivery, Lactate clearance and Organ dysfunction*

Altitude also delays diagnosis, antibiotic administration & evacuation

Initial Management

A. Oxygen: *Correct hypoxia immediately*

B. IV Access: *Two large-bore cannulas*

C. Fluids: Initial Fluid Bolus *(10–20 mL/kg crystalloids cautiously)*

- *Avoid overload in:*
  - *HAPE*
  - *Pulmonary edema*

D. Antibiotics: *Give early broad-spectrum antibiotics* *preferably within first hour*

E. Monitoring: Monitor–MAP, SpO_2, Urine output, Mental status

Septic Shock Algorithm

Suspected infection + hypotension

Assess

Oxygen + IV access

↓

Fluid bolus cautiously

↓

Broad-s

Clinica

Feve

Hypotension

Tachycardia

Tachypnoea

Altered sensorium

YES	NO
Continue monitoring	*Start vasopressor*

↓

Prepare referral/CASEVAC

3. HYPOXIA-RELATED COLLAPSE

Why Collapse Occurs at Altitude

Severe hypoxia may cause:

- *Cerebral hypoperfusion, Syncope, Arrhythmias, Severe pulmonary hypertension, Respiratory failure*

Common Triggers

xertion	nmon

Clinical Features

Severe hypoxia, Cyanosis, Confusion, Exhaustion, Tachypnoea, Altered sensorium, Collapse after exertion

GOLDEN RULE: *"Correct hypoxia first."*

Immediate Actions

High-flow oxygen, Sit patient upright, Warm patient, Restrict exertion, Monitor continuously

If HAPE Suspected then *add Nifedipine & plan descent*

Hypoxia Collapse Algorithm

Collapsed patient at altitude
↓
Check SpO_2 immediately
↓
Severe hypoxia?

YES — High-flow oxygen; Monitor continuously
NO — Evaluate other causes

↓
HAPE/HACE suspected?

YES — Start disease-specific treatment
NO — Continue evaluation

↓
Need evacuation?
↓
Arrange CASEVAC

4. VASOPRESSOR BASICS

When to Start Vasopressors

Use if: Hypotension persists despite fluids, MAP < 65 mmHg, Signs of poor perfusion

Common Vasopressors

Noradrenaline (First-Line Vasopressor)- Dose- 0.05–1 mcg/kg/min IV infusion

Monitoring During Vasopressors

Monitor

Important Precautions

Avoid excessive fluids in HAPE, secure IV access properly, monitor for arrhythmias

Vaspr

Hypote
↓
Fluid responsive?

YES — Continue fluids
↓
Monitor

NO — MAP <65?
↓
Start vasopressor (Noradrenaline)
↓
Continuous monitoring
Prepare ICU referral

Drug Box

Nifedipine	**SR**	**HAPE**

5. SHOCK ALGORITHM

Classification of Shock

olemic	ydration/bleedin

Clinical Features of Shock

Hypotension, Tachycardia, Cold extremities, Altered sensorium, Oliguria, Severe weakness, Cyanosis

Immediate Shock Management

A. ABCDE Assessment

B. Oxygen: *High-flow oxygen*

C. IV Access: *Two large-bore IV lines*

D. Monitoring: ECG, BP, SpO_2, *Urine output*

E. Identify Cause

ɔgenic	nonary edema

Shock Algorithm

Patient collapsed/shocked

↓

ABCDE assessment

High-fl

IV acce

↓

YES **NO**

Assess

Fluid re

YES **NO**

Continue fluids *Start vasopressor*

Monitor closely *ICU referral*

↓

Treat underlying cause

↓

Prepare CASEVAC if unstable

Cardiogenic shock

Severe sepsis

Severe hypoxia

Recurrent collapse

Need for ICU support

Practic

nitor MAP, urine output & treat shock ssively vasopressors early if needed	ion Overhydrate HAPE patients Delay evacuation in unstable patients Miss PE in sudden collapse

Operational Pearls

- "Hypoxia worsens every form of shock."
- "Cold extremities and confusion indicate poor perfusion."
- "Persistent hypotension at altitude is dangerous & Early stabilization improves evacuation survival."

ested reading

vans L, Rhodes A, Alhazzani W, et al. Surviving Sepsis Campaign Guidelines 2021. Intensive Care Med. 021;47(11):1181-1247.

Marino PL. The ICU Book. 4th ed. Philadelphia: Wolters Kluwer; 2014.

anchal AR, Berg KM, Hirsch KG, et al. 2020 AHA Guidelines for Advanced Life Support. Circulation. 020;142(16_suppl_2):S366-S468.

CHAPTER 8: SYNCOPE, SHOCK & COLLAPSE

GOLDEN RULE: COLLAPSE AT ALTITUDE IS SHOCK UNTIL PROVEN OTHERVISE.

1. CARDIAC CAUSES

Why Cardiac Emergencies Increase at Altitude

- Hypoxia → sympathetic activation
- Tachycardia & ↑ myocardial oxygen demand
- Pulmonary hypertension
- Arrhythmogenic stress
- Plaque rupture / thrombosis risk

Common Cardiac Causes of Collapse

Arrhythmias	Palpitations, sudden collapse
STEMI / ACS	Chest pain, ECG changes
Cardiogenic Shock	Hypotension, pulmonary edema
Pulmonary Embolism	Sudden dyspnea, chest pain
Right Ventricular Failure	Raised JVP, severe hypoxia

Cardiac Red Flags

- Chest pain
- Palpitations
- Hypotension
- Syncope during exertion
- Severe hypoxia
- Pulmonary edema
- Sustained arrhythmia
- Shock
- Cold extremities

Immediate Cardiac Assessment

ECG · Pulse · BP · SpO_2 · Capillary · Mental status

Initial Cardiac Stabilization

Oxygen · ECG Monitoring · IV Access · Treat Arrhythmias · STEMI Protocol if indicated

CARDIAC COLLAPSE ALGORITHM

Syncope / Collapse
↓
Check Pulse + BP + ECG
↓
Cardiac cause suspected? (ACS / Arrhythmia / PE)

- YES → Stabilize ABCDE → Oxygen + Monitoring → Treat Arrhythmia / ACS (STEMI Protocol)
  - Shock present?
    - YES → Start Shock Management (See Shock Algorthim)
    - NO → Continue monitoring, Identify cause
  - → Prepare Referral / CASEVAC
- NO → Evaluate other causes (Sepsis / Hypoxia / Neuro / Metabolic)

IMMEDIATE REFERRAL / CASEVAC CRITERIA

- Persistent hypotension (MAP < 65 mmHg)
- Vasopressor requirement
- Cardiogenic shock / Pulmonary edema
- Septic shock / Severe sepsis
- Severe hypoxia (SpO_2 < 85%) despite O_2)
- Suspected pulmonary embolism
- Altered sensorium / GCS decline
- Recurrent syncope or collapse
- Need for ICU / Advanced support
- No improvement despite initial management

PRACTICAL PEARLS

- Check ABCDE immediately.
- Give oxygen early – hypoxia worsens shock.
- Measure MAP – target ≥ 65 mmHg.
- Treat the cause – not just the numbers.
- Prepare early – evacuate early – save lives.

DON'T FORGET

- Delay in fluids for septic shock kills.
- Overhydration can worsen HAPE / pulmonary edema.
- Don't miss PE in sudden unexplained collapse.
- Monitor urine output – key marker of perfusion.
- Early escalation saves organs and lives.

2. SEPTIC SHOCK

Why Sepsis is Dangerous at Altitude

- Hypoxia worsens tissue perfusion & organ dysfunction
- Delayed diagnosis, antibiotics & evacuation
- Rapid progression to multi-organ failure

Common Sources of Infection

Pneumonia (fever, cough) · GI Infection (vomiting, diarrhea) · UTI (dysuria, fever) · Skin Infection (cellulitis, wounds)

Clinical Features of Septic Shock

- Fever / hypothermia
- Hypotension
- Tachycardia
- Tachypnea
- Altered sensorium
- Poor urine output
- Cold extremities
- Capillary refill > 3 sec

Initial Management (Septic Shock Bundle)

- **A** Oxygen – correct hypoxia
- **B** IV Access – two large-bore cannulas
- **C** Fluids – 10–20 mL/kg crystalloids (Cautiously – avoid overload in HAPE/pulmonary edema)
- **D** Antibiotics – give early broad-spectrum (Within first hour)
- **E** Monitoring – MAP, SpO_2, urine output, mental status

SEPTIC SHOCK ALGORITHM

Suspected infection + hypotension / poor perfusion
↓
ABCDE Assessment
↓
Oxygen + IV access + Monitor
↓
Fluid bolus 10–20 mL/kg · Broad-spectrum antibiotics
↓
MAP ≥ 65 mmHg?

- YES → Continue monitoring, Treat source of infection
- NO → Start Vasopressor (Noradrenaline) → Prepare Referral / CASEVAC

4. VASOPRESSOR BASICS

When to Start

- Hypotension persists despite adequte adequate fluids
- MAP < 65 mmHg
- Signs of poor perfusion
- Ongoing shock

Common Vasopressors

Drug	Main Action	Use
Noradrenaline	Vasoconstriction (α)	Septic shock (first line)
Dobutamine	Inotrope ($β_1$)	Cardiogenic shock
Adrenaline	Vasopressor + inotrope	Cardiac arrest / Anaphylaxis

Noradrenaline (First Line)

Dose: 0.05 – 1 mcg/kg/min IV infusion
Titrate to maintain MAP ≥ 65 mmHg

Monitoring During Vasopressors

MAP · Heart Rate · Urine Output · SpO_2 / Lactate · Extremity Perfusion · ECG (arrhythmias)

Important Precautions

- Avoid excessive fluids in HAPE / pulmonary edema
- Secure IV access & infusion line
- Monitor for arrhythmias, tachycardia, ischemia
- Titrate to clinical response (not just BP number)

QUICK DRUG REFERENCE

Drug	Dose	Indication
Noradrenaline	0.05–1 mcg/kg/min IV	Septic shock
Dobutamine	2–20 mcg/kg/min IV	Cardiogenic shock
Adrenaline (IV)	1 mg IV (repeat q3–5 min)	Cardiac arrest
Nifedipine (SR)	30 mg PO	HAPE
Dexamethasone	8 mg IV then 4 mg 6 hourly	HACE
Ceftriaxone	1–2 g IV 12 hourly	Sepsis (broad spectrum)

3. HYPOXIA-RELATED COLLAPSE

Why Collapse Occurs at Altitude

- Cerebral hypoperfusion & syncope
- Arrhythmias
- Severe pulmonary hypertension
- Respiratory failure
- Exhaustion, overexertion
- Rapid ascent

Common Triggers

Severe HAPE · HACE · Exertion · Overexertion · Rapid ascent

Clinical Features

- Severe hypoxia
- Cyanosis
- Confusion
- Exhaustion
- Tachypnea
- Altered sensorium
- Collapse after exertion
- Weak pulse

Immediate Management (Correct Hypoxia First)

- ✓ High-flow oxygen
- ✓ Sit patient upright
- ✓ Keep warm
- ✓ Restrict exertion
- ✓ Monitor continuously (SpO_2, HR, BP, RR)
- ✓ Treat underlying cause (HAPE / HACE / others)
- ✓ Plan descent

HYPOXIA COLLAPSE ALGORITHM

Patient collapsed at altitude
↓
Check SpO_2 immediately
↓
Severe hypoxia? (SpO_2 < 80%)

- YES → High-flow oxygen, Sit up – Monitor continuously
- NO → Evaluate other causes (Cardiac / Neuro / (Sepsis / Metabolic)

HAPE / HACE suspected?

- YES → Start specific treatment
  - O_2 + Nifedipine (HAPE)
  - Dexamethasone (HACE)
- YES → Continue evaluation & management

Improving?

- YES → Continue care, Plan descent
- NO → Arrange CASEVAC

VASOPRESSOR ALGORITHM (IF HYPOTENSION PERSISTS)

Hypotension detected
↓
Fluid responsive?

- YES → Continue fluids, Monitor response
- NO → MAP < 65 mmHg?
  - YES → Start Vasopressor (Noradrenaline infusion)
  - YES → Escalate dose / Add inotrope, Seek expert help / ICU

MAP ≥ 65 mmHg?

- YES → Continue vasopressor, Treat underlying cause
- NO → Escalate care, Prepare ICU / CASEVAC

KEY MONITORING PARAMETERS

MAP · SpO_2 · Heart Rate · Respiratory Rate · Urine Output · GCS · Skin Perfusion

5. SHOCK ALGORITHM (OVERALL)

Patient collapsed / in shock
↓
ABCDE Assessment
High-flow Oxygen • IV Access • Monitoring (ECG, BP, SpO_2, RR, Urine)
↓
Hypotension / Poor Perfusion?

- NO → Evaluate other causes (Neuro / Metabolic / etc) Monitor
- YES → Identify Likely Shock Type
  - **SEPTIC**: Fever / Infection, Warm / cold skin, ↑ RR / WCC
  - **CARDIOGENIC**: Pulmonary edema, S3, cold extremities, Low EF / ACS
  - **OBSTRUCTIVE**: PE / Tamponade, JVP ↑, muffled HS, Sudden collapse
  - **HYPOVOLEMIC**: Bleeding / dehydration, Dry mucosa, Tachycardia

Fluid Bolus (10–20 mL/kg) if appropriate
Correct Hypoxia / Treat cause
↓
Improving?

- YES → Continue Treatment, Monitor Closely, Plan Descent
- NO → Start Vasopressor (if MAP < 65 mmHg), Prepare CASEVAC / ICU

CHAPTER 9
HYPOTHERMIA & FROSTBITE

"No one is dead until warm and dead."

Cold injury is a major cause of morbidity and mortality in high-altitude environments. Hypothermia and frostbite may occur rapidly due to:

- *Extreme cold, Wind chill, Wet clothing, Exhaustion, Hypoxia, Poor shelter*

Early recognition and controlled rewarming are essential to prevent irreversible tissue damage and death.

1. CLASSIFICATION

A. HYPOTHERMIA

Definition: *Hypothermia is a core body temperature <35°C caused by excessive heat loss.*

Severity Classification

Clinical Features

r coordination	► *Ataxia, Bradycardia*	► *Respiratory depression & Cardiac arrest*

B. FROSTBITE

Definition: *Frostbite is tissue freezing injury caused by prolonged cold exposure.*

Common sites: Fingers, Toes, Nose, Ears, Cheeks

Classification of Frostbite

?	necrosis/gangre

e waxy skin *s of sensation*	*Hard frozen tissue* *Cyanosis, Gangrene* *Black discoloration*	*Altered sensorium, Loss of consciousness* *Haemorrhagic blisters, Extensive tissue necrosis* *Respiratory depression*

Classification Algorithm

Cold exposed patient

↓

Check temperature + skin findings

↓

Core temp <35°C?

YES	**NO**
Hypothermia	*Evaluate frostbite*
↓	
Assess severity (mild/moderate/severe)	*Superficial vs deep injury*

2. REWARMING PROTOCOLS

GOLDEN RULE: *"Rewarm gradually and carefully."*

Principles of Rewarming

Prevent Further Heat Loss

Immediately:

Remove wet clothing, dry patient, Insulate from ground, use warm blankets

...e Rewarming	Rewarming
...arm shelter Dry clothes, Warm fluids & Blankets	Warmed IV fluids, warm humidified oxygen External warming devices & Heated blankets

Target Rewarming: *Gradual temperature increase* **&** *avoid rapid aggressive movement*

Important Precautions

Handle gently as rough handling may trigger arrhythmias, avoid direct intense heat and alcohol

Cardiac Monitoring: Continuous ECG monitoring in moderate hypothermia and severe hypothermia

Rewarming Algorithm

Hypothermia diagnosed

↓

Remove wet clothing

Prevent heat loss

↓

YES	NO
Passive warming	Active warming
Warm fluids	Warm IV fluids
Blankets	Warm oxygen

↓

Monitor

YES	NO
Continue warming	ICU referral
	Prepare CASEVAC

3. COLD INJURY MANAGEMENT

Frostbite Management Principles

DO NOT THAW IF: *Refreezing risk exists* **as** *repeated freeze-thaw causes severe tissue damage.*

Rewarming of Frostbite

Rapid Rewarming Technique: *Immerse affected part in warm water 37–39°C for 15–30 minutes but during rewarming expect severe pain, red-purple discoloration and swelling*

Analgesia: Ibuprofen– 400–600 mg PO OR **opioids if severe pain**

Wound Care

After Rewarming

Dry sterile dressings, separate digits with gauze, elevate limb, avoid pressure

Blister Management

Hydration: *Maintain adequate hydration, warm oral/IV fluids*

Infection Prevention: *Consider antibiotics if there is secondary infection, cellulitis, open wounds*

Severe Frostbite *may require thrombolysis, surgical consultation & ICU care*

Frostbite Management Algorithm

Cold injury suspected
↓
Frozen tissue present?

YES
Suspect

Risk of refreezing?

YES NO
Delay t
Protect

Pain control + dressings
↓
Assess tissue viability
↓
Need referral?
↓
Arrange CASEVAC

REFERRAL CRITERIA

Immediate Referral / CASEVAC Required If:

Core temp <32°C

Altered sensorium/coma

Cardiac instability

Severe frostbite

Failure to improve

Need for ICU support

ıccess ; monitoring, dress wounds properly	ue. Insulation, Monitoring, Warm fluids, Oxygen if needed Rough movement, Pressure on frostbitten areas

Referral Algorithm

Cold injury diagnosed
↓
Assess severity
↓

YES
Active warming
ECG monitoring
Prepare CASEVAC
↓
Transport with ongoing warming

NO
Continue local care
Monitor closely

rug Box

Drug	Dose	Use

Practical Pearls

	DO NOT
nove wet clothing immediately & rewarm graduall p patient insulated	Rub frostbitten tissue or use dry direct heat/fire Allow refreezing after thawing

Operational Pearls

- "Loss of shivering indicates worsening hypothermia."
- "Rough handling may precipitate arrhythmias."
- "Refreezing after thawing worsens tissue loss so warm slowly, monitor continuously, evacuate early."

Brown DJA, Brugger H, Boyd J, Paal P. Accidental hypothermia. N Engl J Med. 2012;367(20):1930–1938.
McIntosh SE, Freer L, Grissom CK, et al. Wilderness Medical Society Frostbite Guidelines. Wilderness Environ Med. 2019;30(4 Suppl): S19–S32.
Auerbach PS, Cushing TA, Harris NS, eds. Auerbach's Wilderness Medicine. 7th ed. Philadelphia: Elsevier; 2017.

CHAPTER 9: HYPOTHERMIA & FROSTBITE

⚠ GOLDEN RULE: NO ONE IS DEAD UNTIL WARM AND DEAD.

1. CLASSIFICATION

A. HYPOTHERMIA

Definition: Core body temperature < 35°C caused by excessive heat loss.

Severity Classification

Severity	Core Temp (°C)	Key Clinical Features
Mild	32 – 35°C	Shivering, tachycardia, cold extremities
Moderate	28 – 32°C	Confusion, ataxia, slurred speech, bradycardia
Severe	< 28°C	Coma, arrhythmias, respiratory depression

Mild Hypothermia (32–35°C)
- Intense shivering
- Cold extremities
- Tachycardia
- Poor coordination

Moderate Hypothermia (28–32°C)
- Confusion
- Slurred speech
- Reduced shivering
- Ataxia
- Bradycardia

Severe Hypothermia (<28°C)
- Unconsciousness
- Fixed pupils
- Ventricular arrhythmias
- Respiratory depression
- Cardiac arrest

B. FROSTBITE

Definition: Tissue freezing injury due to prolonged cold exposure.
Common sites: Fingers, toes, nose, ears, cheeks.

Classification of Frostbite

Degree	Features
Superficial	Numbness, tingling, pale waxy skin
Deep	Blisters, hard tissue, decreased sensation
Severe	Black necrosis / gangrene, loss of tissue

Early Features
- ✓ Numbness
- ✓ Tingling
- ✓ Pale, waxy skin
- ✓ Loss of sensation

Severe Features
- Hemorrhagic blisters
- Hard frozen tissue
- Cyanosis
- Black discoloration
- Gangrene

⚠ Red Flag Signs
- Core temperature < 32°C
- Altered sensorium
- Severe arrhythmias
- Loss of consciousness
- Hemorrhagic blisters
- Extensive tissue necrosis
- Hypotension
- Respiratory depression

CLASSIFICATION ALGORITHM

Cold exposed patient
↓
Check core temperature and skin findings
- Core temp < 35°C → HYPOTHERMIA → Determine severity → Mild 32–35°C / Moderate 28–32°C / Severe < 28°C
- Core temp ≥ 35°C → Evaluate FROSTBITE → Assess depth → Superficial / Deep / Severe

2. REWARMING PROTOCOLS

PRINCIPLES

- Prevent further heat loss
- Rewarm gradually and safely
- Handle gently
- Monitor continuously
- Avoid alcohol & direct heat

A. MILD HYPOTHERMIA (32–35°C)

Passive Rewarming
- Warm shelter
- Dry clothes
- Warm sweet fluids
- Warm blankets
- Rest & monitor

B. MODERATE – SEVERE HYPOTHERMIA (≤32°C)

Active Rewarming
- Remove wet clothing
- Warm IV fluids 32–42°C
- Warm humidified oxygen
- External warming devices
- Heated blankets

!
- Handle patient gently – rough handling may trigger arrhythmias
- Avoid rapid aggressive rewarming
- Avoid direct intense heat (fire, heater, hot packs on skin)
- Do not rub or massage the patient
- Monitor ECG in moderate and severe hypothermia

REWARMING ALGORITHM

Hypothermia diagnosed
↓
Remove wet clothing • Dry patient • Insulate from ground
↓
Mild hypothermia (32–35°C)?
- YES → Passive rewarming (shelter, dry clothes, blankets, warm fluids)
- NO (Moderate–Severe) → Active rewarming (warm IV fluids, warm O_2, external warming devices)

Monitor temperature + ECG + vitals
↓
Improving?
- YES → Continue warming and monitoring
- NO → Reassess, check for complications → ICU referral / CASEVAC

3. COLD INJURY MANAGEMENT (FROSTBITE)

Management Principles

✗ **DO NOT THAW** if refreezing risk exists.
Repeated freeze–thaw causes severe tissue damage.

During Rewarming
- Expect severe pain
- Red–purple discoloration
- Swelling
- Numbness
- Do not stop rewarming

Analgesia
Ibuprofen 400–600 mg PO
OR
Opioids if severe pain

Rewarming Technique
Rapid rewarming by immersing affected part in warm water 37–39°C for 15–30 minutes.

After Rewarming – Wound Care
- Dry sterile dressings
- Separate digits with sterile gauze
- Elevate affected limb
- Avoid pressure or tight bandages

Hydration & Nutrition
- Adequate hydration
- Warm oral/IV fluids
- High-calorie diet as tolerated

Infection Prevention
- Clean wound
- Consider antibiotics if:
  - Cellulitis
  - Open wounds
  - Secondary infection

Severe Frostbite – May require
- Thrombolysis (early cases)
- Specialist consultation
- Surgical debridement
- Amputation (if non-viable)

FROSTBITE MANAGEMENT ALGORITHM

Cold injury suspected
↓
Frozen tissue present?
- NO → Evaluate other causes
- YES → Risk of refreezing?
  - YES (High risk) → Do NOT thaw. Protect from further cold exposure
  - NO (Safe to thaw) → Rapid rewarming in 37–39°C water bath 15–30 minutes
    ↓
    Pain control • dressings
    Elevation • hydration
    ↓
    Assess tissue viability
    ↓
    Severe injury?
    - NO → Continue care. Monitor closely
    - YES → Specialist referral / CASEVAC

4. REFERRAL CRITERIA

IMMEDIATE REFERRAL / CASEVAC IF:
- Core temperature < 32°C
- Severe hypothermia (≤28°C)
- Ventricular arrhythmias
- Altered sensorium / coma
- Cardiac instability
- Severe frostbite (deep / advanced)
- Hemorrhagic blisters
- Tissue necrosis / gangrene
- Failure to improve despite treatment
- Need for ICU or specialist care

Before Referral – Stabilize First
- ✓ Rewarm and insulate
- ✓ High-flow oxygen if needed
- ✓ Secure IV access
- ✓ ECG monitoring
- ✓ Treat pain
- ✓ Protect frostbite properly

5. VASOPRESSOR BASICS (FOR SHOCK STATE)

When to Start Vasopressors
- Hypotension persists after adequate fluid resuscitation
- MAP < 65 mmHg
- Signs of poor perfusion
- Cardiogenic / septic shock

Common Vasopressors

Drug	Dose (IV infusion)	Main Use
Norepinephrine (Norepinephrine)	0.05 – 1 mcg/kg/min	Septic shock (most common)
Dobutamine	2 – 20 mcg/kg/min	Cardiogenic shock (low output)
Edreephrine (Adrenaline)	0.01 – 1 mcg/kg/min	Cardiac arrest / Anaphylaxis

Monitoring During Vasopressor Use
- MAP (target ≥ 65)
- Heart Rate (%)
- Urine Output
- Peripheral Perfusion
- Lactate (if available)
- ECG

SHOCK ALGORITHM (OVERALL)

Patient collapsed / in shock
↓
ABCDE Assessment
High-flow O_2 • IV Access • Monitoring (ECG, BP, SpO_2, RR, Urine)
↓
Hypotension / Poor perfusion?
- NO → Evaluate other causes (Neuro, Metabolic, etc.) Continue monitoring
- YES (ngk) → Identify likely shock type
  - SEPTIC: Fever / Infection; Warm / red skin; ↑ RR / WCC / Lactate
  - CARDIOGENIC: Pulmonary edema; Cold extremities; Low EF / ACS
  - OBSTRUCTIVE: PE / Tamponade; PNA / Tension PTX; Sudden collapse
  - HYPOVOLEMIC: Bleeding / dehydration; Dry mucosa; Tachycardia

Fluid Bolus 10–20 mL/kg crystalloids (as appropriate)
↓
Improving?
- YES → Continue treatment. Monitor closely. Plan descent / Referral
- NO → Start Vasopressor (Norepinephrine) MAP target ≥ 65 mmHg

Treat underlying cause • Prepare CASEVAC / ICU

QUICK DRUG REFERENCE

Drug	Dose	Indication
Ibuprofen	400–600 mg PO	Frostbite pain
Warm IV Saline	As needed	Rewarming / shock
Oxygen	High flow	Hypoxia
Morphine	2–5 mg IV	Severe pain

PRACTICAL PEARLS

- Remove wet clothing immediately.
- Loss of shivering – worsening hypothermia.
- Handle gently – rough handling may cause arrhythmias.
- Refreezing after thawing greatly increases tissue loss.
- Rewarm slowly, monitor continuously, evacuate early.

DON'Ts

- ✗ Don't rub or massage cold limbs.
- ✗ Don't use fire / dry direct heat / hot water.
- ✗ Don't allow refreezing after thawing.
- ✗ Don't give alcohol.
- ✗ Don't delay evacuation in severe cases.

KEY MONITORING PARAMETERS

- Core Temp (°C)
- SpO_2 (%)
- Heart Rate (bpm)
- BP / MAP (mmHg)
- Respiratory Rate (/min)
- Urine Output (mL/hr)
- ECG

CHAPTER 10
TRAUMA AT HIGH ALTITUDE

"Trauma plus hypoxia kills rapidly at altitude."

Trauma at high altitude is uniquely dangerous because:

- *Hypoxia worsens shock*
-
-
- *Terrain complicates rescue*
- *Limited resources delay definitive care*

Flail chest
Severe hypoxia
Always assume cervical spine injury until ruled out.

The priorities are:

- *Rapid ABCDE stabilization*
- *Haemorrhage control*
- *Airway and spine protection*
- *Prevention of hypothermia and early evacuation*

1. POLYTRAUMA STABILIZATION

Why Trauma Is More Dangerous at Altitude

Altitude contributes to:

- *Severe hypoxemia, Rapid exhaustion, Hypothermia, Impaired perfusion, Delayed rescue*

Initial Trauma Priorities

GOLDEN RULE: *"Treat life-threatening problems before definitive diagnosis."*

Primary Survey (ABCDE)

A – Airway with Cervical Spine Protection: *Assess: Ability to speak, Airway obstruction, Facial trauma, Blood/vomitus*

B – Breathing: *Assess: Respiratory rate, SpO_2, Chest movement, Air entry, Tracheal deviation*

C – Circulation: *Assess: Pulse, BP, Capillary refill, External bleeding*

D – Disability: *Assess: GCS, Pupils, Limb movement, Focal deficits*

E – Exposure: *Assess for Hidden injuries, Hypothermia, Frostbite*

Prevent

Immedi

Oxygen, Spine stabilisation, IV access × 2, Monitoring, warm patient aggressively

Polytrauma Algorithm

Trauma

ABCDE
↓
Life-threatening injury?

YES NO
Immedi

Oxygen + IV access
Haemorrhage control
Spine protection
↓
Hypotension/hypoxia?
↓
Start shock management
Prepare evacuation

Severe hypoxia
GCS decline
Chest injury

Active bleeding
Respiratory distress

2. HEAD INJURY

Why Head Injury Is Dangerous at Altitude

Hypoxia worsens:

- *Cerebral edema, secondary brain injury, intracranial pressure &*

Common Symptoms

Loss of consciousness
Vomiting
Severe headache
Confusion, Seizures, Amnesia

Flag Signs

SF leak
CS < 13
nequal pupils Recurrent vomiting
eteriorating sensorium
eizures or Focal neurological deficit

Initial Assessment– Check: GCS, Pupils, Limb power, Airway, SpO_2

Immediate Management

Oxygen therapy, Head elevation 30°, Prevent hypotension, avoid hypox

If Raised ICP Suspected

- Signs: Bradycardia, Hypertension, Unequal pupils, GCS decline
- Then: Urgent referral, Airway preparation and ICU care

Seizure Management: Lorazepam (4 mg IV) OR **Midazolam** (5–10 mg IV/IM)

Head Injury Algorithm

Head trauma patient
↓
Assess GCS + pupils
↓
Red flag

YES
Urgent referral — Monitor closely
CT brain if available
↓
Oxygen

GCS wo

YES — NO
Prepare airway — Continue monitoring
ICU/CASEVAC

When to Suspect Spine Injury

Fall from height
Unconscious patient

High-velocity trauma
Head injury with altered sensorium

3. SPINE PRECAUTIONS

GOLDEN RULE: "Assume spine injury in all major trauma."

Immediate Spine Precautions: Manual inline stabilization, cervical collar, log-roll technique, hard board/stretcher

Avoid: Neck flexion/rotation, rough transport, sitting unstable patients upright

Neurological Assessment– Check: Limb movement, sensation, reflexes, bladder function

Spine Precaution Algorithm

Major trauma patient
↓

YES — NO
Immobilize spine — Continue evaluation
Cervical collar
Log-roll precautions
↓
Neurological deficits?

YES — **NO**
Urgent referral — Continue monitoring

4. DAMAGE CONTROL PRINCIPLES

Definition: *Damage control trauma management focuses on saving life first, controlling bleeding, preventing deterioration, rapid evacuation*

Deadly Triad: *Hypothermia, Acidosis & Coagulopathy* **(Altitude worsens all three.)**

Damage Control Algorithm

Severe trauma patient
↓
Control airway + bleeding
↓
Correct hypoxia
Prevent hypothermia
↓
Hemodynamically unstable?

YES — Damage control resuscitation
NO — Continue stabilization

↓
Rapid evacuation & Definitive care

pelvic binder if needed
B. Correct Hypoxia: High-flow oxygen
C. Prevent Hypothermia: Warm blankets, warm IV fluids, re
wet clothing
D. Limited Fluids: Avoid excessive crystalloids, use permiss

5. TRAU

ize First	During Transport
way secure, Oxygen ongoing, controlled bleeding, immobilized, IV access secured, warm the patient	Continue: Oxygen, Monitoring, Spine precautions, Warmth Avoid: Delays, rough handling, unnecessary movement

Trauma Evacuation Algorithm

Trauma stabilized
↓
Need higher center care?

YES
Prepare

Airway secured, Bleeding controlled & Spine immobilized
↓
Continuous monitoring during transport
↓
Early trauma center handover

Indications for Immediate CASEVAC

- **Polytrauma**
- **Severe head injury or spine injury**
- **Chest trauma or Pelvic fracture**
- **Internal bleeding suspected**
- **Need for surgery**

Practical Pearls

ıtrol bleeding rapidly & evacuate early	Delay evacuation in severe trauma

Operational Pearls

- *"Hypoxia worsens traumatic brain injury."*
- *"Cold trauma patients deteriorate rapidly."*
- *"Bleeding control saves more lives than imaging."*
- *"Early evacuation improves survival in mountain trauma."*

ested reading

American College of Surgeons. ATLS Student Course Manual. 10th ed. Chicago: ACS; 2018.
Butler FK, Holcomb JB, Shackelford S, et al. Tactical Combat Casualty Care Guidelines. J Spec Oper Med. 2017;17(2):8–86.
NAEMT. Prehospital Trauma Life Support (PHTLS). 9th ed. Burlington: Jones & Bartlett; 2018.

CHAPTER 10: TRAUMA AT HIGH ALTITUDE

GOLDEN RULE: TREAT LIFE-THREATENING PROBLEMS BEFORE DEFINITIVE DIAGNOSIS.

TRAUMA + HYPOXIA = RAPID DETERIORATION

1. POLYTRAUMA STABILIZATION

Why Trauma Worse at Altitude

- Severe hypoxia
- Hypothermia
- Coagulopathy
- Exhaustion
- Delayed evacuation
- Difficult terrain

Immediate Actions

- High-flow Oxygen
- IV Access ×2 (large bore)
- Monitor: ECG, BP, SpO_2
- Control Hemorrhage
- Spine Precautions
- Prevent Hypothermia

Polytrauma Red Flags

- Hypotension (SBP < 90 mmHg)
- Severe hypoxia (SpO_2 < 90%)
- GCS < 13 or deteriorating
- Chest injury / respiratory distress
- Pelvic instability
- Long bone fractures
- Active bleeding
- Altered consciousness

Primary Survey: ABCDE

A — Airway with cervical spine protection
- Check patency, voice, obstruction, blood/vomit
- Assume C-spine injury until ruled out

B — Breathing
- RR, SpO_2, chest movement, air entry
- Look for: tension PTX, hemothorax, flail chest

C — Circulation
- Pulse, BP, capillary refill, skin
- Control external bleeding immediately

D — Disability (Neurological)
- GCS, pupils, limb movement, signs of deficit

E — Exposure / Environment
- Fully expose, look for hidden injuries
- Prevent heat loss – remove wet clothes, warm blankets

Secondary Survey (Head-to-Toe)

- History (AMPLE: Allergies, Meds, PMH, Last meal, Events)
- Head, Neck (C-spine), Chest, Abdomen, Pelvis, Spine, Limbs
- Vital signs, pain score, urine output
- Investigations as available (FAST, X-ray, Labs)

POLYTRAUMA STABILIZATION ALGORITHM

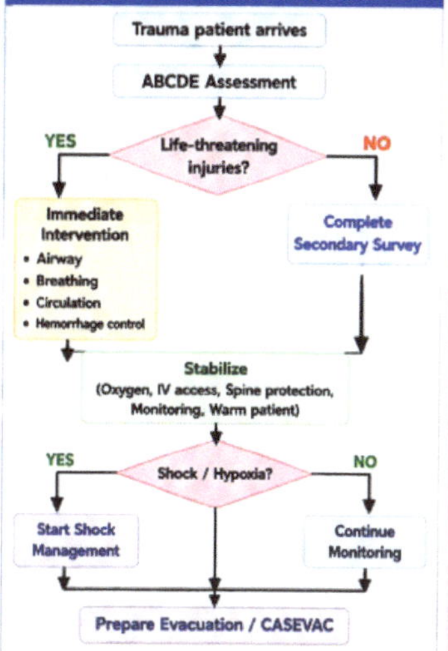

POLYTRAUMA KEY POINTS

- Maintain Spine Protection
- Control bleeding first
- Correct hypoxia early
- Prevent hypothermia
- Reassess continuously

HEMORRHAGE CONTROL

- Direct pressure
- Pressure dressing
- Tourniquet (life-threatening limb bleed)
- Pelvic binder (if pelvic fracture + instability)

Avoid

- ✖ Neck flexion / rotation
- ✖ Rough transport
- ✖ Sitting unstable patient upright
- ✖ Unnecessary movement

2. HEAD INJURY

Common Symptoms

- Loss of consciousness
- Headache
- Vomiting
- Confusion
- Amnesia
- Seizures

Red Flag Signs

- GCS < 13
- Unequal pupils
- Recurrent vomiting
- Seizures
- Focal neurological deficit
- Deteriorating sensorium
- CSF leak (ear/nose)
- Severe headache

Initial Assessment

- GCS
- Pupils
- Limb power
- Airway
- SpO_2, BP, HR

Immediate Management

- ✔ High-flow oxygen
- ✔ Head elevation 30°
- ✔ Maintain normotension
- ✔ Avoid hypoxia & hypercarbia
- ✔ Spine precautions
- ✔ Analgesia
- ✔ Monitor GCS, pupils, vitals

Seizure Management

Lorazepam 4 mg IV

OR

Midazolam 5–10 mg IV/IM

Raised ICP Signs (Brace's Triad)

Hypertension · Bradycardia · Unequal pupils

If ICP Raised / GCS Decline

- Secure airway
- Avoid hypotension
- Urgent evacuation
- CT brain if available

HEAD INJURY ALGORITHM

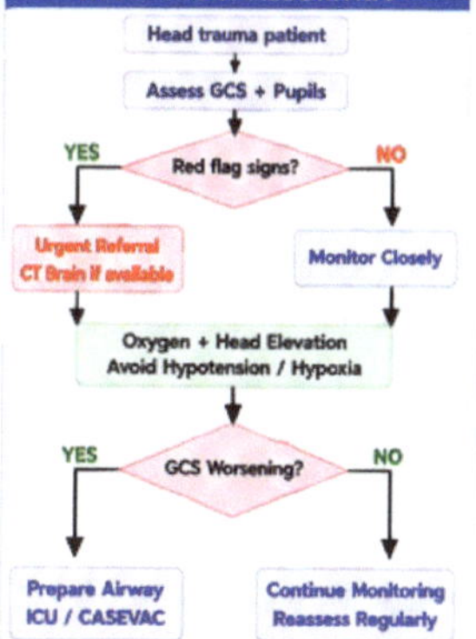

3. SPINE PRECAUTIONS

When to Suspect Spine Injury

- Fall from height
- Unconscious / altered sensorium
- Neck or back pain
- Limb weakness / numbness
- High-velocity trauma
- Head injury
- Distracting injuries

Immediate Spine Precautions

- ✔ Manual inline stabilization
- ✔ Cervical collar
- ✔ Log-roll technique
- ✔ Hard board / Spine board
- ✔ Secure during transport
- ✔ Avoid neck flexion/rotation

Neurological Assessment

Check motor power, sensation, reflexes, and bladder function.

Avoid

- ✖ Neck flexion / rotation
- ✖ Rough transport
- ✖ Sitting unstable patient upright
- ✖ Unnecessary movement

SPINE PRECAUTION ALGORITHM

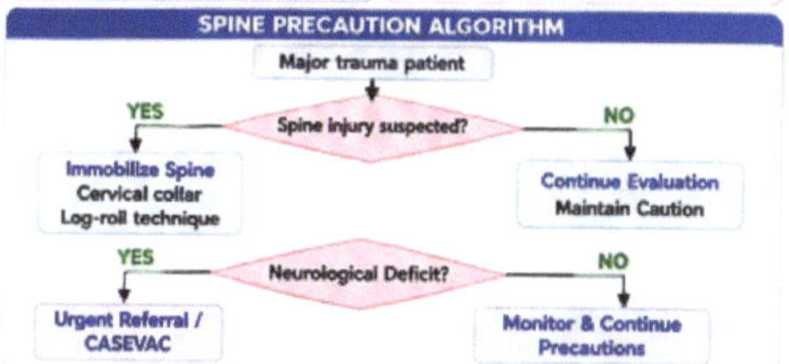

4. DAMAGE CONTROL PRINCIPLES

Goal: Save life first – control bleeding – prevent deterioration – rapid evacuation.

The Deadly Triad

- Hypothermia
- Acidosis
- Coagulopathy

Key Principles

- **A — Control Hemorrhage** (Pressure, dressing, tourniquet, pelvic binder)
- **B — Correct Hypoxia** (High-flow oxygen)
- **C — Prevent Hypothermia** (Remove wet clothes, warm blankets, warm IV fluids)
- **D — Limited Fluids (Permissive Hypotension)** Avoid excessive crystalloids. Use permissive hypotension if no head injury
- **E — Rapid Evacuation – Definitive care** as soon as possible

DAMAGE CONTROL ALGORITHM

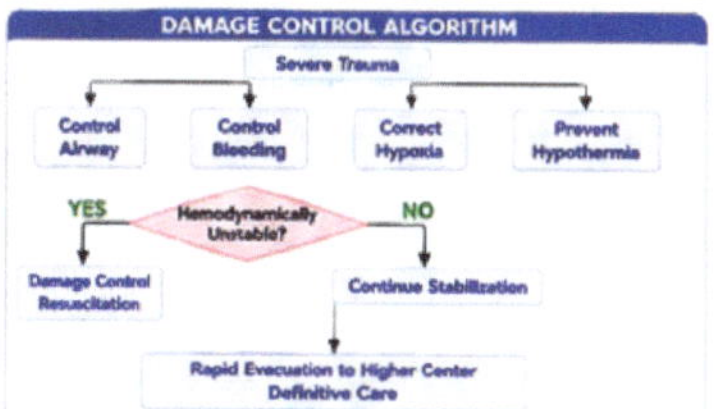

5. TRAUMA EVACUATION

Indications for Immediate CASEVAC

- Polytrauma
- Severe head injury
- Spine injury
- Persistent hypotension (SBP < 90)
- Severe hypoxia (SpO_2 < 90%)
- Chest trauma (PTX, hemothorax, flail chest)
- Pelvic fracture
- Internal bleeding suspected
- Need for surgery / ICU care
- GCS decline / neurological deficit

Before Evacuation – Stabilize First

- Airway secure
- Oxygen ongoing
- Spine–immobilized
- Bleeding controlled
- IV access secured
- Warm patient

TRAUMA EVACUATION ALGORITHM

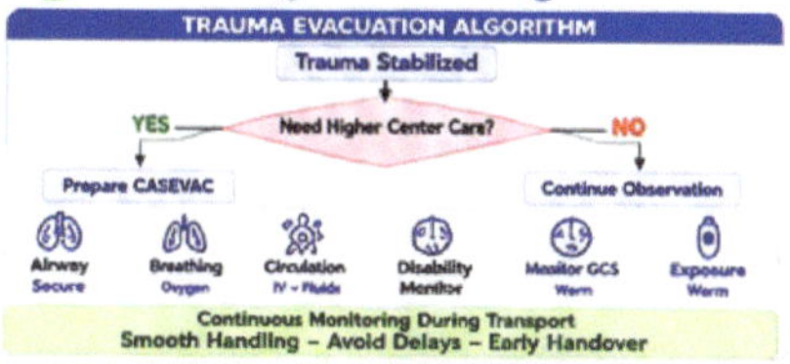

MONITORING CHECKLIST

Parameter	Frequency
SpO_2	Continuous
Heart Rate	Continuous
Blood Pressure	Continuous
Respiatory Rate	Every 5 min
GCS	Every 15 min
Urine Output	Hourly
Temperature	Every 15 min

QUICK DRUG REFERENCE

Drug	Dose	Use
Oxygen	High Flow	Hypoxia
Tranexamic Acid	1 g IV over 10 min then 1 g over 8 h	Major trauma (bleeding)
Lorazepam	4 mg IV	Seizures
Midazolam	5–10 mg IV/IM	Seizures
Fentanyl	25–50 mcg IV	Pain
Normal Saline (warm)	As needed	Fluids / Shock

DO NOT FORGET

- ✖ Delay hemorrhage control
- ✖ Ignore hypoxia
- ✖ Move unstable spine patients
- ✖ Overload fluids in chest trauma
- ✖ Delay evacuation in severe trauma
- ✖ Allow hypothermia to worsen

PRACTICAL PEARLS

- ✔ Prioritize ABCDE every time
- ✔ Control bleeding – it kills faster than hypoxia
- ✔ Hypoxia worsens brain injury and shock
- ✔ Cold trauma patients deteriorate rapidly
- ✔ Reassess frequently

OPERATIONAL PEARLS

- ★ Assume spine injury in all significant trauma
- ★ Manage the patient, not the X-ray
- ★ Damage control first, definitive care later
- ★ Keep patient warm, oxygenated, and perfused
- ★ Plan evacuation early

KEY EQUIPMENT

Oxygen Source · Spine Board · Tourniquet · Pressure Dressings · IV Fluids & Lines · Monitoring Devices

CALL EARLY
EVACUATE EARLY
SAVE LIVES

CHAPTER 11
EMERGENCY DRUG PROTOCOLS

"In high-altitude emergencies, drugs buy time — oxygen, stabilization, and evacuation save lives."

This chapter provides quick-use emergency drug protocols for frontline high-altitude care. Doses are adult doses unless stated otherwise. Adjust for age, weight, renal/hepatic dysfunction, pregnancy, comorbidities, and local pr

Persistent hypotension
fter initial fluid resuscitation
MAP <65 mmHg
Cold extremities/poor
rfusion, oliguria
Altered sensorium due to
ock
Cardiogenic or septic shock

1. VASOPRESSORS

For adult septic shock, norepinephrine is recommended as the first-line vasopressor.

Basic Vasopressor Rules

Moni
Prefe
Correct hypoxia first and use infusion pump for medications whenever possible
Give cautious fluids before vasopressor unless pulmonary edema/cardiogenic shock

Vasopressor Quick Table

renaline / inephrine	*0.05–1 mcg/kg/min IV infusion*	*Septic shock, vasodilatory shock*	*xtravasation, ischemia*
ressin	*0.03 units/min IV infusion*	*Add-on in septic shock*	*chemia, hyponatremia*

Noradrenaline Protocol

tions		***Target***	***Monitoring***
ptic shock *rsistent hypotension* *spite fluids* *isodilatory shock* *ock with MAP <65* *mHg*	*art:* ***0.05*** ***g/kg/min*** *rate every 2–5* *n* *ual range:* ***0.05-*** ***ncg/kg/min***	• *MAP ≥65 mmHg* • *Improved sensorium* • *Warm peripheries* • *Urine output >0.5 mL/kg/hr*	• *BP every 2–5 min initially* • *ECG* • *Urine output* • *Limb perfusion* • *IV site*

Dobutamine Protocol

tions	***Dose***	
rdiogenic shock *w cardiac output* *st-MI pump failure*	• *Start:* ***2–5 mcg/kg/min*** • *Titrate up to* ***20 mcg/kg/min***	*Severe hypotension without vasopressor support* *Uncontrolled tachyarrhythmia*

Adrenaline Protocol

V/IO every 3–5 *uring CPR, as per AHA cardiac arrest algorithm*	***0.5 mg IM*** *of 1:1000 solution* *Repeat every 5–15 min if neec*	• ***0.01–0.5 mcg/kg/min IV infusion***

Vasopressor Algorithm

Shock patient
↓
ABCDE + high-flow oxygen + IV access
↓
MAP <65 mmHg or poor perfusion?
↓
Give cautious crystalloid bolus if appropriate
↓
Fluid responsive?

YES	NO
Continue fluids	Start noradrenaline
Monitor	Titrate to MAP ≥65

↓
Cardiogenic shock/low output?
↓
Add dobutamine if needed
↓
Prepare ICU/CASEVAC

2. SEDATIVES

Golden Rule: "Sedation at altitude can worsen hypoxia – use the lowest effective dose."

Sedativ

-
- Agitation
- Procedural sedation
- Intubation & ventilated patients
- Severe anxiety interfering with oxygen therapy

Always give oxygen
Monitor SpO_2, BP, RR, GCS
Keep airway equipment ready

Sedative Quick Table

ɔam	) mg IV slow	zure, spasm	Long sedation
nyl	i0 mcg IV increments	algesia, trauma, intubation	Respiratory depression

Midazolam Protocol

'e	Agitation / Sedation	Watch For
5–10 mg IM/IV	• **1–2 mg IV slowly** • Repeat cautiously	Respiratory depression Hypotension or worsening hypoxia

3. ANTIEPILEPTICS

First Priority in Seizure

Protect airway, give oxygen, check glucose, prevent injury, give benzodiazepine if ongoing

Seizure Protocol

Step 1 – First 5 Minutes: Airway positioning, Oxygen, Suction, Check glucose & if hypoglycaemia: Dextrose 25 g IV

Step 2 – Benzodiazepine: Lorazepam 4 mg IV slowly, repeat once after 5–10 min if needed OR Midazolam (5–10 mg IM/IV)

Step 3 – Second-Line AED: Levetiracetam: 20–60 mg/kg IV (Common adult dose: **1–3 g IV,** Infuse over 10–15 min) OR **Valproate (20–40 mg/kg IV,** Avoid in liver disease, thrombocytopenia, pregnancy) OR **Phenytoin (20 mg/kg IV,** Rate: max **50 mg/min,** Continuous ECG monitoring)

Antiepileptic Quick Table

iracetam	0–60 mg/kg IV	nd-line, safe pro	Renal adjustment

Status Epilepticus Algorithm

Seizure >5 minutes
↓
Airway + oxygen + glucose check
↓
Lorazepam 4 mg IV
OR Midazolam 5–10 mg IM/IV
↓
Seizure persists?

YES NO
Levetiracetam Monitor
20–60 mg/kg IV Treat cause
↓
Still seizing?
↓
Valproate / Phenytoin
↓
Refractory status
↓
Intubation + ICU + CASEVAC

4. THROMBOLYTICS

Uses in This Handbook

Thrombolytics may be relevant for:

- STEMI when PCI is not immediately available
- Massive pulmonary embolism with shock
- Selected severe frostbite cases under specialist guidance

AHA adult cardiac arrest guidance retains antiarrhythmics such as amiodarone/lidocaine for VF/pVT; thrombolysis is not routine in arrest except selected causes such as suspected pulmonary thrombosis.

STEMI Thrombolysis

Indication

- STEMI diagnosed by ECG
- Symptom onset usually within 6 hours
- PCI not available within acceptable timeline & no contraindication

70–79 k	40 mg IV bolus

Common STEMI Thrombolytics

teplase	Weight-based IV bolus	Preferred where available

Streptokinase Dose

- **1.5 million IU IV over 60 min**

wn malignant intracranial neoplasm emic stroke within 3 months pected aortic dissection ive bleeding nificant closed-head/facial trauma within 3 s	Recent internal bleeding Pregnancy Current anticoagulant use Traumatic CPR Peptic ulcer disease

Post-Thrombolysis Monitoring

Monitor chest pain relief, ST resolution at 60–90 min, reperfusion arrhythmias, bleeding, BP, Neurological status

Failed Thrombolysis

Suspect if:

- Persistent chest pain, <50% ST resolution at 60–90 min, Hemodynamic instability

Action:

- Urgent rescue PCI / CASEVAC

5. EMERGENCY INFUSIONS

General Infusion Safety

Use infusion pump whenever possible

Labe

Ment

Monitor vitals continuously

Avoid calculation errors in low-light/high-stress settings

Emergency Infusion Quick Table

renaline	0.05–1 mcg/kg/min	hock
ose 25 g	IV bolus	ypoglycaemia
esium sulphate	2 g IV over 10–20 min	orsades/eclampsia

Amiodarone Protocol

VF/pVT Cardiac Arrest

- **300 mg IV/IO bolus** then second dose: **150 mg IV/IO** (This matches AHA adult cardiac arrest drug dosing)

Stable Wide-Complex Tachycardia

- **150 mg IV over 10 min** then infusion if needed

Bradycardia Protocol

- **Atropine- 1 mg IV** (repeat every 3–5 min, maximum **3 mg**
- **If ineffective then** Dopamine infusion, Adrenaline infusion **or** Transcutaneous pacing

Hypoglycaemia Protocol

- **If conscious then give** oral glucose if safe
- **If unconscious / unable to swallow then give 25 g IV dextrose** (Example: 50 mL of 50% dextrose then start dextrose-containing fluids if recurrent

Severe Symptomatic Hyponatremia

- **Indications:** *Seizure, coma, severe confusion, severe neurological symptoms*
- **3% Saline: 100 mL IV over 10 min,** *repeat up to 2 more times if severe symptoms persist*
- **Correction Limit:** *Avoid overcorrection, usual maximum:* **8–10 mEq/L in 24 hours**

DKA Insulin Infusion

- **Before giving Insulin,** check potassium *if normal then start* **regular Insulin (0.1 units/kg/hr IV infusion)**
- *If glucose falls <200 mg/dL: Add dextrose AND continue insulin until anion gap closes*

Tranexamic Acid in Trauma

- **Indication:** *Major trauma with suspected significant bleeding, best within 3 hours of injury*
- **Dose: 1 g IV over 10 min,** *Then* **1 g IV over 8 hours**

Emergency Drug Safety Checklist

Before
Corr
Contraindications checked, Monitoring available

High-Altitude Drug Pearls

noradrenaline early in persistent shock	Give aggressive fluids in HAPE/cardiogenic shock
at seizures rapidly	Delay benzodiazepines in active seizure
nitor ECG during antiarrhythmics and ressors	Thrombolysis without checking contraindications
pare evacuation for all unstable patients	Run unlabelled infusions

Operational Pearls

- *"Oxygen is the first emergency drug at altitude."*
- *"Vasopressors support perfusion; they do not treat the cause."*
- *"Sedation without airway planning is dangerous."*
- *"Thrombolysis saves myocardium but can kill if contraindications are missed."*
- *"Every infusion must be labelled, monitored, and reassessed."*

sted reading:

arino PL. The ICU Book. 4th ed. Philadelphia: Wolters Kluwer; 2014.

merican Heart Association. ACLS Provider Manual. Dallas: AHA; 2020.

oint Formulary Committee. British National Formulary (BNF). London: BMJ Group and Pharmaceutical Press; 024.

oberts JR, Custalow CB, Thomsen TW. Roberts and Hedges' Clinical Procedures in Emergency Medicine. 7th ed. hiladelphia: Elsevier; 2018.

EPINEPHRINE (ADRENALINE)

Life-Saving Drug – Vasopressor • Bronchodilator • Cardiac Stimulant

DRUG CLASS
Catecholamine
Non-selective α and β adrenergic agonist

1. PHARMACOLOGY

- **Mechanism:**
  - α1: Vasoconstriction → ↑ SVR, ↑ BP
  - β1: ↑ Heart rate, ↑ Contractility, ↑ CO
  - β2: Bronchodilation, ↓ Mediator release, ↓ Airway edema
- **Onset:** 1–2 minutes (IV)
- **Peak:** 2–5 minutes
- **Duration:** 5–20 minutes
- **Metabolism:** COMT, MAO
- **Elimination:** Renal
- **Half-life:** ~2–3 minutes

2. INDICATIONS

- **CARDIAC**
  - Cardiac arrest (as per ACLS)
  - Symptomatic bradycardia (refractory)
  - Refractory shock
  - Anaphylaxis (first line)
- **RESPIRATORY**
  - Severe bronchospasm
  - Croup (nebulization)
- **OTHER**
  - Add-on in septic/cardiogenic shock
  - Local hemostasis (with local anesthetic)

3. CONTRAINDICATIONS / CAUTIONS

Absolute: None in life-threatening situations

Use Caution:
- Tachyarrhythmias
- Severe hypertension
- Ischemic heart disease
- Pheochromocytoma
- Hyperthyroidism
- Diabetes mellitus
- Narrow angle glaucoma (nebulization)
- Extravasation risk (IV infusion)

4. DOSAGE & ADMINISTRATION

INDICATION	ROUTE	DOSE (ADULT)	REPEAT / NOTES
Cardiac Arrest	IV/IO	1 mg (1 mL of 1:1000)	Every 3–5 min during CPR
Anaphylaxis	IM (anterolateral thigh)	0.5 mg (0.5 mL of 1:1000)	Repeat every 5–15 min if needed
Severe Bronchospasm	Nebulization	2.5 mg (2.5 mL of 1:1000)	Dilute in 2.5 mL NS; nebulize
Refractory Shock	IV Infusion	0.01–0.5 mcg/kg/min	Titrate to effect (MAP ≥ 65 mmHg)
Bradycardia (refractory)	IV	0.5 mg (0.5 mL of 1:1000)	Repeat every 3–5 min
Local Hemostasis	Infiltration	0.5–1 mL of 1:1000	Mix with local anesthetic

5. PREPARATION OF STANDARD SOLUTION

Stock Ampoule: Epinephrine 1 mg/mL (1:1000)
1 mL = 1 mg

Dilution for Infusion (Recommended)
Add 1 mL (1 mg) Epinephrine (1:1000)
to 99 mL 0.9% Normal Saline (NS)
Total volume = 100 mL
Concentration = 10 mcg/mL

6. INFUSION PREPARATION (WITHOUT INFUSION PUMP)

Make solution as above: **1 mg in 100 mL NS = 10 mcg/mL**

DOSE REQUIRED (mcg/kg/min)	CALCULATION GUIDE (For 70 kg patient) Dose (mcg/min)	mL/hr of solution (10 mcg/mL)	Approx. drops/min* (20 gtt/mL set)
0.01	0.7	4 mL/hr	1–2 drops/min
0.02	1.4	8 mL/hr	2 drops/min
0.05	3.5	21 mL/hr	5–7 drops/min
0.10	7	42 mL/hr	10–14 drops/min
0.20	14	84 mL/hr	20–28 drops/min
0.30	21	126 mL/hr	30–42 drops/min
0.50	35	210 mL/hr	50–70 drops/min

*Drop factor may vary (15–20 gtt/mL). Adjust as per set used.
Always monitor BP and titrate.

7. DOSE TITRATION ALGORITHM (INFUSION)

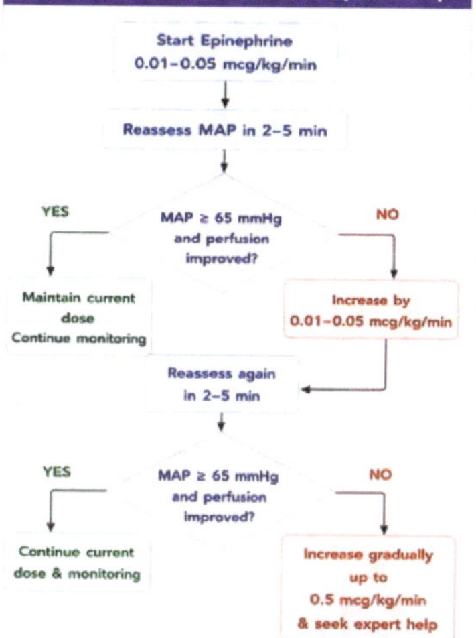

8. SPECIAL ADMINISTRATION NOTES

IV BOLUS (CARDIAC ARREST)
Give rapidly via IV/IO.
Flush with 10–20 mL NS after each dose.

IM (ANAPHYLAXIS)
Inject in mid-outer thigh.
Do not give IV for anaphylaxis unless in arrest.

NEBULIZATION (BRONCHOSPASM)
Dilute 2.5 mL (1:1000) in 2.5 mL NS and nebulize.

INFUSION
Use infusion pump if available.
If not available, use drop method as per table and monitor closely.

EXTRAVASATION RISK
Stop infusion immediately.
Treat with phentolamine (5–10 mg diluted in 5–10 mL NS) infiltrated area.

9. ADVERSE EFFECTS

COMMON
- Tachycardia
- Palpitations
- Tremors
- Headache
- Anxiety
- Pallor

SERIOUS
- Arrhythmias
- Hypertension
- Myocardial ischemia
- Peripheral ischemia / digital necrosis
- Extravasation injury
- Pulmonary edema

10. MONITORING

- BP (invasive if possible) – every 2–5 min
- ECG – continuous
- SpO_2 – continuous
- Urine output – hourly
- Peripheral perfusion, skin color, capillary refill
- Look for signs of extravasation
- Mental status

11. COMPATIBILITY

Compatible with:
- 0.9% NaCl (Normal Saline)
- 5% Dextrose

Do not mix with:
- Sodium bicarbonate
- Phenytoin
- Hydroxocobalamin

Flush line before and after infusion.

12. KEY POINTS

- ✓ Epinephrine is a first-line drug in cardiac arrest and anaphylaxis.
- ✓ Use the lowest effective dose.
- ✓ Titrate infusion to maintain MAP ≥ 65 mmHg.
- ✓ Monitor closely for arrhythmias and extravasation.
- ✓ Oxygen, fluids and treat underlying cause.

13. STORAGE

- Store below 25°C.
- Protect from light.
- Do not freeze.
- Use within 24 hours after dilution.

14. QUICK REFERENCE

Cardiac Arrest (IV/IO)	1 mg every 3–5 min
Anaphylaxis (IM)	0.5 mg repeat 5–15 min
Shock (Infusion)	0.01–0.5 mcg/kg/min
Bronchospasm (Neb)	2.5 mg in 2.5 mL NS

REMEMBER
RIGHT DRUG
RIGHT DOSE
RIGHT ROUTE
RIGHT TIME
SAVES LIVES

⚠ Always give oxygen • Correct hypoxia and acidosis • Reassess frequently • Early evacuation when indicated

NORADRENALINE (NOREPINEPHRINE)

Potent α-adrenergic agonist – First line vasopressor for shock

1. PHARMACOLOGY

- **Class:** Vasopressor
- **Mechanism:** Potent alpha-1 agonist >> beta-1 agonist
- **Action:** Vasoconstriction (arterioles & veins)
  - → ↑ Systemic vascular resistance
  - → ↑ Blood pressure & coronary perfusion
- **Onset:** 1–2 minutes
- **Peak:** 5–10 minutes
- **Duration:** Continuous infusion dependent
- **Metabolism:** COMT & MAO
- **Elimination:** Renal

2. INDICATIONS

- Septic shock (first line)
- Vasodilatory shock
- Persistent hypotension after adequate fluid resuscitation
- Neurogenic shock
- Cardiogenic shock with hypotension
- Peri-arrest hypotension
- MAP < 65 mmHg despite fluids

3. CONTRAINDICATIONS / CAUTIONS

- Hypovolemia (relative – correct first)
- Severe peripheral vascular disease
- Extravasation risk (local necrosis)
- Severe tachyarrhythmias (use with caution)
- Hypertrophic obstructive cardiomyopathy
- Use via central line if possible
- CAUTION in:
  - Ischemic heart disease
  - Elderly
  - Severe liver impairment

4. DOSAGE & ADMINISTRATION

Route	Starting Dose	Usual Dose Range	Maximum Dose
IV Infusion	0.05 mcg/kg/min	0.05 – 1.0 mcg/kg/min	1.0 mcg/kg/min

Titration: Increase by 0.01–0.05 mcg/kg/min every 2–5 min

Target: MAP ≥ 65 mmHg, improved perfusion, urine output > 0.5 mL/kg/hr

5. MONITORING

- BP (invasive if available) – every 2–5 min initially
- ECG – continuous
- SpO_2 – continuous
- Urine output – hourly
- Limb perfusion, skin color, capillary refill
- Look for signs of extravasation (pain, blanching, swelling)

6. PREPARATION OF INFUSION

A. STANDARD PREPARATION (RECOMMENDED)

1. **Dilution:** 4 mg (4 mL) of Noradrenaline (1 mg/mL) in 100 mL 5% Dextrose or Normal Saline
2. **Concentration:** 40 mcg/mL

CALCULATION GUIDE (For 40 mcg/mL solution)

Dose (mcg/kg/min)	Drops/min* (60 gtt/mL)	mL/hr	For 70 kg patient (mcg/min)
0.05	5	5	3.5
0.10	10	10	7
0.20	20	20	14
0.30	30	30	21
0.50	50	50	35
1.00	100	100	70

*If using 20 drops/mL set, mL/hr = Drops/min ÷ 20

B. HIGHER CONCENTRATION (For low rate requirement)

1. **Dilution:** 4 mg (4 mL) in 50 mL NS/D5
2. **Concentration:** 80 mcg/mL

Use separate calculation: Dose (mcg/kg/min) × weight (kg) ÷ 80 = mL/hr

IMPORTANT POINTS

- Use infusion pump if available – safer and more accurate.
- Use central line if possible.
- Label the syringe/bottle: Drug, concentration, dose, time.
- Change infusion every 24 hours.
- Protect from light.

WITHOUT INFUSION PUMP – HOW TO SET MANUALLY

1. Use the standard preparation (4 mg in 100 mL = 40 mcg/mL).
2. Calculate required mL/hr from table (or formula).
3. If using macrodrip set (20 drops/mL):

   Drops/min = mL/hr × 20

4. Adjust roller clamp to get the calculated drops/min.
5. Check BP every 5 min and adjust as needed.

⚠ Never run noradrenaline via unmonitored peripheral line.

7. DOSE TITRATION ALGORITHM

Start Noradrenaline 0.05 mcg/kg/min

↓

Reassess MAP in 2–5 min

↓

MAP ≥ 65 mmHg & Perfusion Improved?

- YES → Maintain current dose → Continue monitoring
- NO → Increase by 0.01–0.05 mcg/kg/min → Reassess again in 2–5 min

↓

MAP ≥ 65 mmHg?

- YES → Continue titration & monitoring
- NO → Increase gradually up to max 1 mcg/kg/min

↓

If inadequate response at max dose:

- Reassess volume status
- Check for other causes
- Add second vasopressor
- Consider ICU / advanced care

8. ADVERSE EFFECTS

COMMON

- Hypertension
- Reflex bradycardia
- Headache
- Pallor
- Anxiety

SERIOUS

- Arrhythmias
- Myocardial ischemia
- Peripheral ischemia / digital necrosis
- Extravasation injury
- Tissue necrosis
- Sudden BP fluctuations

9. EXTRAVASATION MANAGEMENT

1. Stop infusion immediately.
2. Do not remove the IV cannula.
3. Aspirate any residual drug.
4. Elevate the limb.
5. Apply warm compress.
6. Consider Phentolamine: 5–10 mg diluted in 5–10 mL NS infiltrated area (by slow injection).
7. Surgical consult if severe.

10. COMPATIBILITY

Compatible: NS, D5W

Do not mix with: Sodium bicarbonate, Hydroxycobalamin, Phenytoin.

Flush line before and after infusion.

11. SPECIAL SITUATIONS

- **Septic Shock:** First line vasopressor → target MAP ≥ 65 mmHg.
- **Cardiogenic Shock with hypotension:** Use with inotrope (e.g., Dobutamine)
- if low cardiac output.
- **Neurogenic Shock:** Maintain adequate preload, then use noradrenaline.
- **Peri-arrest hypotension:** Use during CPR to maintain coronary perfusion.
- **Pregnancy:** Use only if benefit outweighs risk.
- **Pediatrics:** 0.05–1 mcg/kg/min (titrate as per response).

12. KEY FORMULAS

- Dose (mcg/min) = Dose (mcg/kg/min) × Weight (kg)
- mL/hr (40 mcg/mL) = Dose (mcg/kg/min) × Weight (kg) ÷ 40
- Drops/min (60 gtt/mL) = mL/hr × 60
- If 20 gtt/mL set: Drops/min = mL/hr × 20

13. STORAGE

- Store below 25°C.
- Protect from light.
- Use within 24 hours after preparation.

QUICK REFERENCE

START	TARGET	MAX DOSE	ONSET	PEAK
0.05 mcg/kg/min	MAP ≥ 65 mmHg	1 mcg/kg/min	1–2 min	5–10 min

REMEMBER

- Right Drug
- Right Dose
- Right Route
- Right Patient
- Monitor & Reassess

LIFE-SAVING PEARLS

- ✓ Noradrenaline is the FIRST-LINE vasopressor in most shock states.
- ✓ Always correct hypoxia and volume status first.
- ✓ Titrate slowly and reassess frequently.
- ✓ Monitor for extravasation every few minutes.
- ✓ Early goal-directed therapy saves lives.

RIGHT DRUG
RIGHT DOSE
RIGHT TIME
SAVES LIVES

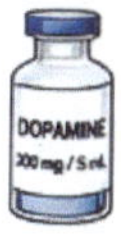

Strength:

Strength:
40 mg/mL
(200 mg / 5 mL)

DOPAMINE

Catecholamine Inotrope / Vasopressor

Increases cardiac output, blood pressure and renal perfusion

DRUG CLASS

Sympathomimetic
Catecholamine

1. PHARMACOLOGY

- **Mechanism:** Stimulates D_1, β_1 and α_1 adrenergic receptors in a dose-dependent manner.
- **Onset (IV):** 2–5 minutes
- **Peak effect:** 5–10 minutes
- **Duration:** 5–20 minutes (while infusion continues)
- **Half-life:** ~2 minutes
- **Metabolism:** Metabolized by MAO & COMT
- **Elimination:** Renal (metabolites)
- **Route:** IV infusion only (via central or peripheral line)
- **Pregnancy:** Category C (use if benefits > risk)

Dose-dependent effects:

- 1–3 mcg/kg/min: D_1 (renal/mesenteric vasodilation)
- 3–10 mcg/kg/min: β_1 (↑ HR, ↑ contractility)
- >10 mcg/kg/min: α_1 (vasoconstriction ↑ BP)

2. INDICATIONS

- Cardiogenic shock
- Acute decompensated heart failure (low cardiac output)
- Bradycardia with hypotension
- Hypotension during anesthesia
- Renal hypoperfusion (to improve urine output)
- Vasodilatory shock (adjunct) (e.g., septic shock with low SVR)

3. CONTRAINDICATIONS / CAUTIONS

Absolute Contraindications

- Pheochromocytoma
- Hypersensitivity to dopamine

Use Caution

- Tachyarrhythmias
- Ischemic heart disease
- Hypertension
- Peripheral vascular disease
- Extravasation (risk of tissue necrosis)
- Elderly and patients with renal impairment
- Do not mix with bicarbonate solutions (risk of inactivation)

4. DOSAGE & ADMINISTRATION (IV INFUSION)

DOSE	EFFECT	INDICATION / USE
1 – 3 mcg/kg/min	D_1 (renal, mesenteric vasodilation) ↑ Renal blood flow, ↑ urine output	Renal protection (low urine output) Early shock states
3 – 10 mcg/kg/min	β_1 (↑ HR, ↑ contractility) ↑ Cardiac output	Cardiogenic shock Heart failure Bradycardia with hypotension
> 10 mcg/kg/min	α_1 (vasoconstriction) ↑ SVR, ↑ BP	Severe hypotension (vasodilatory shock, refractory shock)

Administration Notes

- Start at the lowest effective dose and titrate to response.
- Use infusion pump for accurate delivery.
- Monitor BP, HR, ECG, urine output and peripheral perfusion.

5. PREPARATION

Standard Preparation

- Add 200 mg (5 mL) dopamine to 245 mL of 5% Dextrose (Total volume = 250 mL) Concentration = 800 mcg/mL
- (0.8 mg/mL)

(or)

Add 400 mg (10 mL) dopamine to 245 mL of 5% Dextrose Concentration = 1600 mcg/mL (1.6 mg/mL)

Preferred Diluent

- 5% Dextrose in Water (D5W) (Do NOT use Normal Saline)

Stability

- 24 hours at room temperature

6. ADMINISTRATION NOTES

- Infuse via central line if possible. Peripheral line may be used for short term at low doses (< 10 mcg/kg/min).
- Titrate dose every 5–15 minutes based on clinical response.
- Do not mix with bicarbonate or alkaline solutions.
- Avoid extravasation. If occurs: stop infusion, elevate limb, apply warm compress.

7. ADVERSE EFFECTS

Common

- Tachycardia, palpitations
- Arrhythmias
- Nausea, vomiting
- Headache
- Anxiety

Serious

- Hypertension (at high doses)
- Myocardial ischemia
- Peripheral vasoconstriction
- Tissue necrosis (extravasation)
- Renal ischemia (high doses)
- Arrhythmias (VT, VF, AF)

Monitor closely. Use the lowest effective dose.

8. MONITORING

- Continuous ECG monitoring
- Blood pressure (invasive if available)
- Heart rate and rhythm
- Urine output (target > 0.5 mL/kg/hr)
- Peripheral perfusion (skin, cap refill, pulses)
- Serum electrolytes
- Signs of extravasation
- Daily weight & fluid balance

9. IMPORTANT POINTS

- ✓ Dopamine is a potent inotrope and vasopressor.
- ✓ Dose-dependent effects – titrate carefully.
- ✓ Use D5W only – do NOT use NS.
- ✓ Taper down gradually – do not stop abruptly.
- ✓ Monitor for arrhythmias and ischemia.
- ✓ Maintain adequate volume status.
- ✓ Protect from light.

10. COMPATIBILITY / INCOMPATIBILITY

Compatible with:

- 5% Dextrose (D5W)
- Heparin (at low concentration)

Do NOT mix with:

- ✗ Sodium Bicarbonate
- ✗ Normal Saline
- ✗ Other alkaline solutions
- ✗ Blood products

11. STORAGE

- Store at room temperature (15–30°C).
- Protect from light.
- Do not freeze.
- Use within 24 hours after preparation.

12. QUICK REFERENCE DOSE TABLE

CONDITION	INITIAL DOSE	TITRATION
Cardiogenic Shock / Heart Failure	3 – 5 mcg/kg/min	Increase by 2.5–5 mcg/kg/min every 5–15 min
Renal Hypoperfusion (Low Urine Output)	1 – 3 mcg/kg/min	Titrate to urine output > 0.5 mL/kg/hr
Bradycardia with Hypotension	3 – 10 mcg/kg/min	Adjust to maintain BP and HR
Severe Hypotension (Vasodilatory Shock)	> 10 mcg/kg/min	Titrate to maintain MAP and perfusion

REMEMBER
RIGHT DRUG • RIGHT DOSE • RIGHT ROUTE
RIGHT TIME • RIGHT PATIENT
SAVE LIVES

EMERGENCY PEARL
Start low and go slow.
Titrate to clinical response and perfusion.
Monitor closely – dopamine can be powerful but risky.

TITRATE CAREFULLY • MONITOR CONTINUOUSLY • DOCUMENT RESPONSE

DOBUTAMINE

Strength:
250 mg / 20 mL
(12.5 mg/mL)

Synthetic Catecholamine Inotrope

Increases myocardial contractility and cardiac output

DRUG CLASS
Inotropic Agent
Sympathomimetic

1. PHARMACOLOGY

- **Mechanism:** Stimulates β_1-adrenergic receptors predominantly → increases myocardial contractility (positive inotrope) and stroke volume → ↑ cardiac output.
- **Onset (IV):** 1–2 minutes
- **Peak effect:** 5–10 minutes
- **Duration:** While infusion continues
- **Half-life:** ~2 minutes
- **Metabolism:** Minimal; conjugated in liver
- **Elimination:** Renal (metabolites)
- **Route:** IV infusion (preferably via central line)
- **Pregnancy:** Category C (use if benefits > risk)

2. INDICATIONS

- Acute decompensated heart failure with low cardiac output
- Cardiogenic shock (with hypotension and evidence of low output)
- Post-cardiac surgery or myocarditis with poor LV function
- Low cardiac output states not responding to volume resuscitation
- Adjunct in certain cardiac procedures requiring increased CO

3. CONTRAINDICATIONS / CAUTIONS

Contraindications

- Hypertrophic obstructive cardiomyopathy (HOCM)
- Hypersensitivity to dobutamine
- Tachyarrhythmias not controlled

Use Caution

- Hypotension (may worsen if volume depleted)
- Severe valvular stenosis
- Ischemic heart disease
- Renal or hepatic impairment
- Elderly and critically ill patients
- Extravasation (risk of tissue necrosis) – use central line if possible

4. DOSAGE & ADMINISTRATION (IV INFUSION ONLY)

INDICATION / USE	STARTING DOSE	TITRATION	MAXIMUM DOSE
General Use	2.5–5 mcg/kg/min		20 mcg/kg/min
Cardiogenic Shock / Low Output	5 mcg/kg/min	Increase by 2.5 mcg/kg/min every 10–15 min based on response	20 mcg/kg/min
Acute Heart Failure (Low Output)	2.5 mcg/kg/min		20 mcg/kg/min

Administration Notes

- Use infusion pump for accurate delivery.
- Prefer central venous line for administration. Peripheral line may be used short term at low doses (< 5 mcg/kg/min).
- Titrate to clinical response: ↑ cardiac output, ↑ urine output, improved perfusion, stable BP.

5. PREPARATION

Standard Concentration
250 mg Dobutamine in 250 mL 5% Dextrose (D5W)
= 1 mg/mL (1000 mcg/mL)
OR
250 mg Dobutamine in 500 mL D5W = 0.5 mg/mL (500 mcg/mL)

Preparation Steps

- Add 250 mg (20 mL of 12.5 mg/mL) dobutamine to D5W.
- Gently mix.
- Label concentration and time.
- Do not mix with other medications.

Stability

- 24 hours at room temperature.

6. ADMINISTRATION NOTES

- Infuse via central line if possible.
- Peripheral line may be used for short term at low doses (< 5 mcg/kg/min).
- Titrate every 10–15 minutes to desired hemodynamic effect.
- Do not mix with sodium bicarbonate or alkaline solutions.
- Protect from light.

7. ADVERSE EFFECTS

Common

- Tachycardia, palpitations
- Arrhythmias (PVCs, SVT, AF)
- Hypotension
- Headache
- Nausea, vomiting
- Tremors

Serious

- Ventricular arrhythmias
- Myocardial ischemia
- Severe hypotension
- Extravasation (tissue necrosis)

Monitor closely. Use the lowest effective dose.

8. MONITORING

- Continuous ECG monitoring
- Blood pressure (invasive if available)
- Urine output (target > 0.5 mL/kg/hr)
- Serum electrolytes (K^+, Mg^{2+})
- Signs of ischemia (ECG changes, chest pain)
- Daily weight & fluid balance

9. IMPORTANT POINTS

- ✓ Dobutamine increases cardiac output without significantly increasing preload.
- ✓ Dose-dependent effects – titrate to response.
- ✓ Wean gradually when discontinuing to avoid rebound decline in cardiac output.
- ✓ Ensure adequate volume status before starting.
- ✓ Avoid extravasation – stop infusion immediately if swelling, pain, or redness occurs.
- ✓ Monitor for arrhythmias and ischemia.

10. COMPATIBILITY / INCOMPATIBILITY

Compatible with:

- 5% Dextrose (D5W)
- Heparin (at low concentration)

Do NOT mix with:

- Sodium Bicarbonate
- Other alkaline solutions
- Blood products

Flush line with D5W before and after.

11. STORAGE

- Store at room temperature (15–30°C).
- Protect from light.
- Do not freeze.
- Use within 24 hours after preparation.

12. QUICK REFERENCE DOSE TABLE

INDICATION	STARTING DOSE	TITRATION	MAX DOSE
General Use	2.5–5 mcg/kg/min	↑ 2.5 mcg/kg/min every 10–15 min	20 mcg/kg/min
Cardiogenic Shock / Low Output	5 mcg/kg/min	↑ 2.5 mcg/kg/min every 10–15 min	20 mcg/kg/min
Acute Heart Failure (Low Output)	2.5 mcg/kg/min	↑ 2.5 mcg/kg/min every 10–15 min	20 mcg/kg/min

13. REMEMBER

RIGHT DRUG
RIGHT DOSE
RIGHT ROUTE
RIGHT TIME
RIGHT PATIENT
SAVE LIVES

14. EMERGENCY PEARLS

- ★ Start low and go slow.
- ★ Titrate to clinical response – not heart rate alone.
- ★ Dobutamine improves contractility; may cause tachycardia.
- ★ Discontinue gradually.
- ★ Monitor closely for arrhythmias and ischemia.

TITRATE CAREFULLY • MONITOR CONTINUOUSLY • DOCUMENT RESPONSE

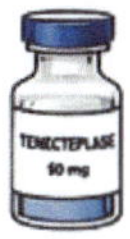

TENECTEPLASE

(Recombinant Tissue Plasminogen Activator – TNK-tPA)

Thrombolytic Agent – For Acute Myocardial Infarction (STEMI)

DRUG CLASS

Thrombolytic / Fibrinolytic (tPA)

1. PHARMACOLOGY

- **Mechanism:** Binds to fibrin and converts plasminogen to plasmin → breaks down fibrin clot (fibrinolysis).
- **Onset:** Within minutes
- **Peak effect:** 30–90 minutes
- **Half-life:** 20–24 minutes
- **Metabolism:** Not applicable (protein)
- **Elimination:** By liver (proteolytic cleavage)
- **Route:** IV bolus
- **Pregnancy:** Category B (use if benefits > risk)
- **Appearance:** White to off-white lyophilized powder

2. INDICATIONS

- ST-Elevation Myocardial Infarction (STEMI) when PCI is not available within 120 minutes of first medical contact.
- Cardiogenic shock due to STEMI (if no immediate PCI).
- Symptom onset ≤ 12 hours. (Greatest benefit within 3 hours).

3. CONTRAINDICATIONS / CAUTIONS

ABSOLUTE CONTRAINDICATIONS

- Any prior intracranial hemorrhage
- Known structural cerebral vascular lesion
- Known malignant intracranial neoplasm
- Ischemic stroke within 3 months (except acute ischemic stroke within 4.5 h and no hemorrhage on CT)
- Suspected aortic dissection
- Active internal bleeding
- Significant closed-head or facial trauma within 3 months
- Intracranial or intraspinal surgery within 2 months

RELATIVE CONTRAINDICATIONS (Use with caution)

- History of hypertension
- Age > 75 years
- Remote stroke (> 3 months)
- Recent major surgery or trauma (< 3 weeks)
- Pregnancy, peptic ulcer disease, diabetic retinopathy

4. DOSSE & ADMINISTRATION

INDICATION	DOSE (IV BOLUS)	MAXIMUM DOSE	NOTES
STEMI	Single IV bolus based on body weight (not infusion)	50 mg	Give as IV bolus over 5–10 seconds

WEIGHT-BASED DOSING

Body Weight (kg)	Dose (mg)	Body Weight (kg)	Dose (mg)
< 60	30	80 – 89	45
60 – 69	35	≥ 90	50
70 – 79	40		

Use actual body weight. Round dose to nearest 5 mg.

5. PREPARATION (IV BOLUS)

Reconstitution

- Add 5 mL of Sterile Water for Injection to the 50 mg vial of Tenecteplase.
- Gently swirl – DO NOT SHAKE.
- Final concentration = 10 mg/mL.

Administration

- Withdraw the required dose as per weight (see table in section 4).
- Administer as IV bolus over 5–10 seconds.
- Flush line with 10 mL NS after bolus.

Do not mix with any other drug.

6. ADMINISTRATION NOTES

- Give as early as possible (door-to-needle time should be minimal).
- Ensure patient is on continuous cardiac monitoring.
- Do not use the same IV line for other drugs during and after administration.
- Avoid arterial puncture at non-compressible sites for 24 hours.

7. ADJUNCTIVE THERAPY (Unless contraindicated)

BEFORE / AT THE TIME OF TENECTEPLASE

- **Aspirin:** 150–325 mg PO (chewed) (If not given before)
- **Clopidogrel:** 300 mg PO load (if < 75 yrs and no contraindication)
- **Anticoagulant:** Enoxaparin (preferred) 30 mg IV bolus, then 1 mg/kg SC every 12 h (max 100 mg/dose) for up to 8 days or until PCI OR
- **UFH:** 60 U/kg IV bolus (max 4000 U), then 12 U/kg/hr infusion (max 1000 U/hr) for 48 h or until PCI

DURING & AFTER

- **Continue Aspirin:** 75–150 mg daily
- **Clopidogrel:** 75 mg daily for at least 12 months
- **Beta blocker, Statin, ACE inhibitor:** as indicated
- **Nitrate, Morphine, Oxygen:** as per need

8. MONITORING

- Continuous ECG monitoring
- Monitor BP, HR, RR, SpO_2 frequently
- Watch for signs of bleeding
- Neurological assessment regularly

Lab monitoring:

- CBC, PT/INR, aPTT (baseline & as indicated)
- Cardiac enzymes (as per protocol)

9. ADVERSE EFFECTS

COMMON

- Minor bleeding (gum, epistaxis, bruising)
- Nausea, vomiting
- Hypotension

SERIOUS

- Major bleeding (GI, GU, intracranial)
- Hemorrhagic stroke
- Allergic / anaphylactoid reactions (rare)
- Reperfusion arrhythmias

Stop drug & initiate appropriate management if major bleeding or stroke occurs.

10. IMPORTANT POINTS

- ✓ Tenecteplase is given as SINGLE IV BOLUS – not an infusion.
- ✓ Maximum benefit if given within 3 hours of symptom onset.
- ✓ Do not give if PCI can be performed within 120 minutes.
- ✓ Ensure no contraindication before administration.
- ✓ Avoid IM injections and unnecessary invasive procedures for 24 hours after administration.
- ✓ Record exact time of administration.

11. DRUG INTERACTIONS

Increased bleeding risk with:

- Anticoagulants (warfarin, heparin, DOACs)
- Antiplatelets (aspirin, clopidogrel, prasugrel, ticagrelor)
- NSAIDs
- SSRIs

Avoid other fibrinolytics or potent anticoagulants within 24 hours.

12. COMPATIBILITY / DILUENT

- Supplied as lyophilized powder in vial (50 mg).
- Reconstitute with 5 mL Sterile Water for Injection (Final concentration = 10 mg/mL).
- Administer IV bolus only.
- Do not mix with other drugs.
- Flush line with 0.9% NS before and after.

13. STORAGE

- Store below 25°C.
- Protect from light.
- Do not freeze.
- Keep vial in original package.
- Use reconstituted solution immediately.

14. KEY POINTS

- ✓ Weight-based single IV bolus.
- ✓ Not an infusion.
- ✓ Early administration saves myocardium & lives.
- ✓ Always combine with antiplatelets & anticoagulants unless contraindicated.

15. QUICK REFERENCE DOSE TABLE (STEMI)

Weight (kg)	Tenecteplase Dose (mg) IV IV Bolus
< 60	30 mg
60 – 69	35 mg
70 – 79	40 mg
80 – 89	45 mg
≥ 90	50 mg

16. REMEMBER

RIGHT DRUG
RIGHT DOSE
RIGHT ROUTE
RIGHT TIME
SAVE MYOCARDIUM
SAVE LIVES

VERIFY CONTRAINDICATIONS • CHECK WEIGHT • CALCULATE DOSE • GIVE ON TIME • MONITOR CLOSELY

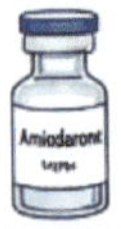

Amiodarone
150 mg / 3 mL
Injection

AMIODARONE

(Antiarrhythmic – Class III)

For life-threatening tachyarrhythmias

DRUG CLASS

Class III Antiarrhythmic
(Potassium channel blocker)
Also has Class I, II & IV effects

1. PHARMACOLOGY

- **Mechanism:** Prolongs phase 3 repolarization by blocking potassium channels → increases action potential duration & refractory period in atrial, ventricular and AV nodal tissue.
- **Onset (IV):** 5–15 minutes
- **Peak effect:** 30–60 minutes
- **Half-life:**
  - Distribution: 1–8 hours
  - Elimination: 20–100 days (accumulates)
- **Metabolism:** Hepatic (CYP3A4)
- **Elimination:** Biliary (70%), Renal (30%)
- **Drug interactions:** Many (see notes)
- **Pregnancy:** Category D
- **Appearance:** Clear, yellow solution

2. INDICATIONS

IV USE

- Ventricular fibrillation (VF) / Pulseless VT (during cardiac arrest – refractory)
- Sustained Ventricular Tachycardia (with pulse)
- Supraventricular tachycardia (e.g., AF with pre-excitation – WPW) when other drugs fail
- Atrial fibrillation / flutter – rate or rhythm control in unstable patients

ORAL (Long term)

- Maintenance of sinus rhythm in AF/flutter
- Recurrent VT suppression

3. CONTRAINDICATIONS / CAUTIONS

Contraindications

- Severe sinus node dysfunction
- Second or third degree AV block (without pacemaker)
- Cardiogenic shock due to bradycardia
- Known hypersensitivity

Use Caution

- Hypotension
- Severe bradycardia
- QT prolongation
- Liver or thyroid dysfunction
- Concomitant drugs causing QT prolongation
- Pregnancy (avoid unless absolutely necessary)

4. DOSAGE & ADMINISTRATION (IV)

INDICATION	DOSE	DILUTION	INFUSION
Pulseless VT / VF (During Cardiac Arrest)	300 mg IV/IO bolus (5 mg/kg) Second dose: 150 mg IV/IO (2.5 mg/kg)	Dilute each dose in 20 mL D5W (Do NOT use NS)	Push over 10 minutes via IV/IO
Stable Wide Complex Tachycardia (Monomorphic VT)	150 mg IV over 10 minutes	Dilute in 100 mL D5W	Infuse over 10 minutes
Atrial Fibrillation / Flutter with RVR	150 mg IV over 10 minutes Then infusion 1 mg/min for 6 hours Then 0.5 mg/min for 18 hours	Dilute in 250 mL D5W	Over 24 hours (as 6 h + 18 h regimen)

Note: Always use D5W for dilution. Do NOT mix with NS or Ringer's Lactate.

5. INFUSION PREPARATION (WITHOUT INFUSION PUMP)

Stock: Amiodarone 150 mg / 3 mL (50 mg/mL)

A. Standard Infusion (for maintenance or after loading)

Add 900 mg (18 mL) amiodarone to 250 mL D5W.
Final concentration = 3.6 mg/mL (≈ 4 mg/mL)

- For 1 mg/min (60 mg/hr):
  60 mg/hr ÷ 4 mg/mL = 15 mL/hr
  Set IV rate to 15 mL/hr (macrodrip 20 gtt/mL)
  = 15 drops/min
- For 0.5 mg/min (30 mg/hr):
  30 mg/hr ÷ 4 mg/mL = 7.5 mL/hr
  Set IV rate to 7–8 drops/min

B. If only 100 mL bottle available

Add 360 mg (7.2 mL) amiodarone to 100 mL D5W.
Final concentration = 3.6 mg/mL

- For 1 mg/min: 15 drops/min
- For 0.5 mg/min: 7–8 drops/min

6. DOSE TITRATION / MAINTENANCE

- After initial bolus, continue infusion as per regimen.
- Reduce dose if:
  - Bradycardia (<50/min)
  - Hypotension (SBP < 90 mmHg)
  - QTc > 500 msec
- Transition to oral maintenance once stable.
- Oral maintenance dose:
  200 mg twice daily for 1 week then 200 mg once daily.

7. DOSE ALGORITHM (ADULT)

CARDIAC ARREST – REFRACTORY VF / pVT

VF/pVT persists after defibrillation & CPR
↓
Amiodarone 300 mg IV/IO over 10 min
↓
If persists
↓
Amiodarone 150 mg IV/IO over 10 min
↓
Continue CPR and treat reversible causes

STABLE VT (WITH PULSE)

Wide complex tachycardia (VT)
↓
Amiodarone 150 mg IV over 10 min
↓
If needed: 1 mg/min for 6 hours
↓
Then 0.5 mg/min for 18 hours
↓
Switch to oral therapy

8. ADVERSE EFFECTS

Common

- Hypotension (during rapid infusion)
- Bradycardia
- Nausea, vomiting
- Phlebitis (IV site)
- Elevated liver enzymes

Serious

- Pulmonary toxicity (fibrosis, pneumonitis)
- Thyroid dysfunction (hypo or hyperthyroidism)
- Hepatotoxicity
- QT prolongation, Torsades de Pointes
- Corneal microdeposits (with long term use)
- Neuropathy, tremors, ataxia
- Skin photosensitivity (blue-gray discoloration)

⚠ **Monitor closely during infusion. May cause life-threatening arrhythmias.**

9. MONITORING

- Continuous ECG monitoring (watch QT interval)
- BP, HR, SpO_2 – frequently
- Liver function tests (baseline & periodic)
- Thyroid function tests (baseline & every 3–6 months for long term)
- Chest X-ray & pulmonary function (if long term therapy)
- Eye exam (if long term)
- IV site for phlebitis/infiltration
- Drug interactions & electrolytes (K^+, Mg^{2+})

10. IMPORTANT NOTES

- ✔ Always dilute in D5W, never in NS or RL.
- ✔ Do not give IV push – always over 10 minutes.
- ✔ Hypotension is common with rapid infusion.
- ✔ Long half-life – adverse effects may appear weeks to months later.
- ✔ Interacts with Warfarin, Digoxin, Beta blockers, CCBs, Statins, many others.
- ✔ Wash hands / protect skin from sunlight in long term use (photosensitivity).

11. DRUG INTERACTIONS (IMPORTANT)

- Increases effect/toxicity of:
  - Warfarin (↑ INR)
  - Digoxin (↑ digoxin levels)
  - Beta blockers, Calcium channel blockers (↑ bradycardia)
  - Statins (↑ myopathy risk)
- Avoid with other QT prolonging drugs:
  - Macrolides, Fluoroquinolones, Antipsychotics, etc.
- CYP3A4 inhibitor – increases levels of many drugs.

12. COMPATIBILITY / DILUENT

Compatible with:

✔ Dextrose 5% (D5W)

Do NOT mix with:

✘ 0.9% Normal Saline (NS)
✘ Ringer's Lactate (RL)

Flush line with D5W before and after administration.

13. STORAGE

- Store below 25°C.
- Protect from light.
- Do not freeze.
- After dilution: Use within 24 hours.

14. ORAL PREPARATION

Tablets: 200 mg
Take with food.
Swallow whole.
Do not crush.

15. QUICK REFERENCE DOSES

SITUATION	DOSE (IV)
Cardiac arrest – refractory VF/pVT	300 mg IV bolus, then 150 mg IV bolus
Stable VT (with pulse)	150 mg IV over 10 min
AF / Flutter with RVR (unstable)	150 mg IV over 10 min then 1 mg/min for 6 h, then 0.5 mg/min for 18 h
Maintenance oral	200 mg PO BID x 1 week, then 200 mg OD

16. REMEMBER

RIGHT DRUG
RIGHT DOSE
RIGHT ROUTE
RIGHT TIME
RIGHT MONITORING

SAVE LIVES

AMIODARONE SAVES LIVES – USE CORRECTLY, DILUTE CORRECTLY, AND MONITOR CLOSELY.

MIDAZOLAM

Short-acting Benzodiazepine

Sedative • Anxiolytic • Anticonvulsant • Amnestic

DRUG CLASS

Benzodiazepine

1. PHARMACOLOGY

- **Mechanism:** Enhances GABA activity at $GABA_A$ receptors → CNS depression
- **Onset:**
  - IV: 1–2 minutes
  - IM: 10–15 minutes
  - IN: 5–10 minutes
- **Peak:**
  - IV: 2–5 minutes
  - IM: 20–30 minutes
- **Duration:** 1–6 hours (dose dependent)
- **Metabolism:** Hepatic (CYP3A4)
- **Elimination half-life:** 1.5–2.5 hours
- **Excretion:** Renal (inactive metabolites)

2. INDICATIONS

- Seizures (acute management)
- Sedation/anxiolysis
- Procedural sedation
- Pre-operative medication
- Induction/maintenance of anesthesia (adjunct)
- ICU sedation (short term)
- Alcohol withdrawal (adjunct)

3. CONTRAINDICATIONS / CAUTIONS

Absolute Contraindications

- Hypersensitivity to benzodiazepines
- Myasthenia gravis (severe)
- Severe respiratory insufficiency without ventilatory support

Use Caution

- Hypotension / shock
- Elderly / debilitated patients
- Hepatic impairment
- Obstructive sleep apnea
- Pregnancy (avoid near delivery)
- Concomitant CNS depressants (opioids, alcohol)

4. DOSAGE & ADMINISTRATION (ADULT)

INDICATION	ROUTE	DOSE
Acute Seizure	IV	2–5 mg IV slowly (over 1–2 min) May repeat 2–5 mg after 5–10 min if needed
	IM (if no IV)	5–10 mg IM
Agitation / Anxiety	IV	1–2 mg IV slowly; repeat as needed
	IM	5–10 mg IM
Procedural Sedation	IV	1–2 mg IV; titrate in 0.5–1 mg increments until adequate sedation (Usual total 1–5 mg)
Pre-operative Medication	IV	1–2 mg IV
	IM	7.5–15 mg IM (30–45 min pre-op)
ICU Sedation (Short Term)	IV Infusion	Start 1–2 mg/hr; titrate to effect (Up to 20 mg/hr may be required)
Alcohol Withdrawal (Adjunct)	IV	2–4 mg IV; repeat as needed (Usual 10–20 mg in first 1–2 hr)

Pediatric: 0.05–0.2 mg/kg IV/IM (Max single dose 5 mg)

5. PREPARATION (IV / IM)

Available Strength
5 mg/mL (1 mL = 5 mg)

Dilution for IV Administration (Recommended)

For slow IV/injection:
Dilute with 0.9% Normal Saline

- **For 2 mg dose:**
  Draw 0.4 mL (2 mg) +
  0.6 mL NS → Total 1 mL
- **For 5 mg dose:**
  Draw 1 mL (5 mg) +
  0 mL NS → Total 1 mL

IM Injection:
May be given undiluted (deep IM)
Preferred site: Upper outer quadrant of gluteal region.

6. INFUSION PREPARATION & ADMINISTRATION (WITHOUT PUMP)

Prepare Standard Infusion:

- Add 10 mg (2 mL of 5 mg/mL) midazolam to 100 mL of 0.9% NS.
- Concentration = 0.1 mg/mL (100 mcg/mL)

Administration (Using Microdrip Set):

Dose Required	mL/hr	Drops/min* (macrodrip 20 gtt/mL)
1 mg/hr	10 mL/hr	3–4
2 mg/hr	20 mL/hr	7–8
5 mg/hr	50 mL/hr	17–18
10 mg/hr	100 mL/hr	33–34

*For microdrip (60 gtt/mL):
Drops/min = mL/hr
(1 mL/hr ≈ 1 drop/min)

Reassess sedation & vitals frequently.

7. ONSET, DURATION & CHARACTERISTICS

ROUTE	ONSET	DURATION	NOTES
IV	1–2 min	1–2 hr	Rapid onset, short duration
IM	10–15 min	2–6 hr	Painful; avoid in small muscle
IN (Intranasal)	5–10 min	1–2 hr	Useful in seizures (0.2 mg/kg)
Infusion (IV)	5–15 min	Infusion dependent	Short-acting; good for ICU

8. DOSE TITRATION ALGORITHM (SEDATION / AGITATION)

Assess patient & indication
Ensure airway & oxygenation
↓
Give Midazolam
(See dose chart above)
↓
Reassess in 2–5 minutes
↓
Adequate sedation achieved?

- YES → Maintain lowest effective dose
  Monitor
- NO → Repeat/Increase dose
  by 0.5–1 mg
  Titrate cautiously

9. ADVERSE EFFECTS

COMMON

- Drowsiness, sedation
- Dizziness
- Hypotension
- Respiratory depression
- Amnesia

SERIOUS

- Respiratory arrest
- Profound hypotension
- Paradoxical agitation (rare)
- Prolonged sedation (esp. elderly/hepatic disease)
- Phlebitis (with IV use)

⚠ **Risk increased with opioids, alcohol, other CNS depressants.**

10. MONITORING

Continuous monitoring of:

- Respiratory rate and effort
- SpO_2
- Blood pressure
- Heart rate
- Level of consciousness (RASS score)
- Sedation depth
- Look for paradoxical reactions

11. REVERSAL

Flumazenil (Benzodiazepine Antagonist)

- Dose: 0.2 mg IV over 15 sec
- May repeat 0.2 mg every 1 min
  (Max total 1 mg)
- Use with caution in chronic benzo users, seizure disorders, or mixed overdose (risk of precipitating seizures).

12. SPECIAL CONSIDERATIONS

- Use the lowest effective dose.
- Titrate slowly, especially in elderly, hepatic dysfunction, or hypovolemic patients.
- Avoid rapid IV bolus in unstable patients.
- Not ideal for long-term ICU sedation (risk of accumulation); prefer ø agent with short half-life and daily sedation breaks.

13. COMPATIBILITY

Compatible with:

- 0.9% NS
- 5% Dextrose

Avoid mixing with:

- Sodium bicarbonate
- Heparin (high concentration solutions)
- Phenytoin (in same line)

Flush line before and after administration.

14. STORAGE

- Store below 25°C.
- Protect from light
- Do not freeze
- Use within 28 days after opening

15. KEY POINTS

- ✓ Short-acting benzodiazepine
- ✓ Rapid onset via IV
- ✓ Useful in seizures, sedation, anxiety
- ✓ Titrate slowly to avoid respiratory depression
- ✓ Always ensure airway & oxygen
- ✓ Monitor closely after each dose

16. QUICK REFERENCE DOSES

INDICATION	DOSE (ADULT)
Seizure (IV)	2–5 mg IV; repeat 2–5 mg
Agitation (IV)	1–2 mg IV
Procedural Sedation	1–2 mg IV (titrate 0.5–1 mg)
Pre-operative (IM)	7.5–15 mg IM
ICU Infusion	1–2 mg/hr

REMEMBER

RIGHT DRUG • RIGHT DOSE • RIGHT ROUTE • RIGHT TIME • MONITOR CLOSELY
SEDATION WITHOUT MONITORING CAN BE DANGEROUS.

SAVE LIVES

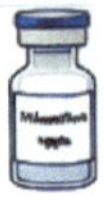

Levetiracetam
500 mg/5 mL
Injection

LEVETIRACETAM

(Antiepileptic)

Broad spectrum antiepileptic • Well tolerated • Minimal drug interactions

DRUG CLASS

Antiepileptic / Anticonvulsant

1. PHARMACOLOGY

- Mechanism: Binds to synaptic vesicle protein 2A (SV2A) → modulates neurotransmitter release
- Onset (IV): 5–15 minutes
- Peak effect: 15–30 minutes
- Duration: 6–8 hours
- Metabolism: Minimal hepatic metabolism
- Elimination: Renal (66% unchanged)
- Half-life: 6–8 hours (normal renal function)
- Protein binding: <10%
- Drug interactions: Minimal
- Pregnancy: Category C (use if benefit > risk)

2. INDICATIONS

- Acute treatment of focal seizures
- Adjunctive therapy in partial onset seizures
- Juvenile myoclonic epilepsy
- Primary generalized tonic-clonic seizures
- Status epilepticus (as 2nd line agent after benzodiazepines)
- Seizure prophylaxis in neurosurgery
- Traumatic brain injury (early seizure prophylaxis)

3. CONTRAINDICATIONS / CAUTIONS

Contraindications

- Hypersensitivity to levetirecetam
- Severe renal impairment without dose adjustment

Use Caution

- Renal impairment (dose adjustment required)
- Pregnancy and lactation
- History of mood or behavioral disorders
- Elderly patients

4. DOSAGE & ADMINISTRATION

INDICATION	ROUTE	ADULT DOSE	COMMENTS
Acute Seizure / Status Epilepticus	IV	20–60 mg/kg (Max 4,500 mg)	Give over 10–15 min (See dosing table below)
Adjunctive Therapy	PO / IV	500 mg – 1,500 mg twice daily	Titrate based on response (Max 3,000 mg/day)
Seizure Prophylaxis (Neurosurgery / TBI)	PO / IV	500 mg – 1,000 mg twice daily	Start pre-op or as early as possible
Pediatric (Seizure)	IV / PO	20–60 mg/kg twice daily	Max 3,000 mg/day

In status epilepticus: If seizure persists after first dose (20–60 mg/kg), a second dose 10–20 mg/kg may be given after 10–15 minutes.

5. PREPARATION (IV)

Available Strength: 500 mg/5 mL (100 mg/mL)

How to Prepare IV Infusion

Calculate required dose (mg) → Draw volume from ampoule → Dilute in 100 mL of 0.9% Normal Saline (NS).

Final concentration = (Dose in mg) / 100 mL (mg/mL)

Infuse over 10–15 minutes using infusion set.

Example:

If dose required = 1,000 mg
Draw 10 mL (1,000 mg) from ampoule
Add to 100 mL NS → Concentration = 10 mg/mL
Infuse over 10–15 minutes.

6. IV DOSE CALCULATION GUIDE (ACUTE / STATUS)

Recommended dose: 20–60 mg/kg (Max 4,500 mg)
Dilute required dose in 100 mL NS and infuse over 10–15 min

WEIGHT (kg)	DOSE RANGE (mg)		VOLUME TO WITHDRAW (From 100 mg/mL ampoule)	
	20 mg/kg	60 mg/kg	20 mg/kg	60 mg/kg
20	400 mg	1,200 mg	4 mL	12 mL
30	600 mg	1,800 mg	6 mL	18 mL
40	800 mg	2,400 mg	8 mL	24 mL
50	1,000 mg	3,000 mg	10 mL	30 mL
60	1,200 mg	3,600 mg	12 mL	36 mL
70	1,400 mg	4,200 mg	14 mL	42 mL
≥75	1,500 mg*	4,500 mg (Max)	15 mL	45 mL

*Maximum recommended single dose = 4,500 mg.

7. ADMINISTRATION

IV Infusion (Preferred in Acute Seizure)

- Infuse over 10–15 minutes.
- Use infusion pump if available.
- Flush line with NS before and after.

IV Push (If Infusion Not Possible)

- Dilute in at least 10 mL NS.
- Inject slowly over 2–3 minutes.
- Follow with NS flush.

Oral Administration

- Tablets: 250 mg, 500 mg, 750 mg, 1,000 mg
- Can be taken with or without food.

8. ADVERSE EFFECTS

Common (Usually mild)

- Drowsiness
- Dizziness
- Fatigue
- Headache
- Irritability / mood changes
- Nasopharyngitis
- Loss of appetite

Serious (Uncommon)

- Behavioral changes (agitation, depression, hostility)
- Suicidal thoughts / ideation
- Severe skin reactions (SJS, TEN)
- Blood dyscrasias (rare)

Stop drug & seek medical help if severe mood changes or rash occur.

9. MONITORING

- Neurological status
- Seizure frequency
- Renal function (BUN, Serum Creatinine)
- Behavior / mood changes
- CBC (if long term use)

10. RENAL DOSE ADJUSTMENT

Creatinine Clearance (mL/min)	Dose Adjustment
≥ 80	No adjustment
50 – 79	500 mg – 1,000 mg every 12 hours
30 – 49	250 mg – 750 mg every 12 hours
< 30	250 mg – 500 mg every 12 hours
On Dialysis	250 mg – 500 mg every 24 hours (+ extra 250–500 mg after dialysis)

11. COMPATIBILITY / DILUENT

Compatible with:

- 0.9% Normal Saline (NS)
- 5% Dextrose (D5W)

Do NOT mix with:

- Ringer's Lactate
- Dextrose solutions containing calcium (e.g., D5NS with Ca)

Flush line before and after administration.

12. STORAGE

- Store below 25°C.
- Protect from light.
- Do not freeze.
- Use within 28 days after opening ampoule.

13. KEY POINTS

- ✓ Safe, effective, and well tolerated
- ✓ Minimal drug interactions
- ✓ Ideal for status epilepticus
- ✓ Renal adjustment is essential
- ✓ Can be given IV or orally

14. DRUG INTERACTIONS

Minimal clinically significant drug interactions.

Does not induce or inhibit hepatic enzymes.

15. QUICK REFERENCE DOSES

INDICATION	ADULT DOSE (IV unless specified)
Acute Seizure / Status Epilepticus	20–60 mg/kg (Max 4,500 mg) over 10–15 min
Adjunctive Therapy	500–1,500 mg twice daily (PO or IV)
Seizure Prophylaxis (Neurosurgery / TBI)	500–1,000 mg twice daily (PO or IV)

REMEMBER
Treat the patient, not just the seizure.

RIGHT DRUG • RIGHT DOSE • RIGHT ROUTE • RIGHT TIME
Seizure control saves brain. Act fast, act safe.

SEIZURE CONTROL SAVES LIVES

Concentration
3 g NaCl / 100 mL
= 513 mEq/L

3% SALINE (HYPERTONIC SALINE)

Hyperosmolar Agent – Reduces Intracranial Pressure

Also used in Hyponatremia

DRUG CLASS
Hyperosmolar Solution
Electrolyte

1. PHARMACOLOGY

- **Mechanism:** Creates an osmotic gradient across the blood-brain barrier → draws water out of brain parenchyma → reduces cerebral edema and intracranial pressure (ICP).
- **Onset:** Within 5–15 minutes
- **Peak effect:** 30–60 minutes
- **Duration:** 2–4 hours
- **Metabolism:** Not metabolized
- **Elimination:** Renal excretion
- **Half-life:** Effect lasts 2–4 hours
- **Pregnancy:** Category C (use if benefits outweigh risks)
- **Route:** IV infusion (peripheral or central)

2. INDICATIONS

- Raised Intracranial Pressure (due to trauma, ICH, tumor, post-op)
- Cerebral Edema
- Impending or established cerebral herniation (as temporizing therapy)
- Symptomatic Hyponatremia (acute or severe)

3. CONTRAINDICATIONS / CAUTIONS

Contraindications
- Severe renal failure / anuria
- Severe congestive heart failure / fluid overload
- Hypernatremia
- Dehydration / hypovolemia

Use Caution
- Elderly
- Liver failure
- SIADH (risk of overcorrection)
- Central pontine myelinolysis risk in chronic hyponatremia (correct slowly)

4. DOSAGE & ADMINISTRATION

INDICATION	DOSE	ADMINISTRATION	NOTES
Raised ICP (Adults)	2–5 mL/kg IV bolus (Max 250 mL)	Infuse over 10–20 minutes	May repeat 1–2 times if needed Assess response clinically or by ICP
Raised ICP (Pediatrics)	2–5 mL/kg IV bolus (Max 250 mL)	Infuse over 10–20 minutes	Repeat based on clinical response and serum sodium
Symptomatic Hyponatremia (Adults)	100 mL IV bolus over 10 minutes (May repeat up to 2–3 times)	Then infusion 0.5–1 mL/kg/hr	Aim: ↑ Na^+ by 4–6 mEq/L in first 6 hours
Symptomatic Hyponatremia (Pediatrics)	2–5 mL/kg IV bolus over 10–20 min	Then infusion 0.5–1 mL/kg/hr	Do not increase Na^+ by > 8–10 mEq/L in 24 hr

Always monitor serum sodium and osmolality closely.

5. PREPARATION & ADMINISTRATION

Available Solution

3% Sodium Chloride (NaCl)
= 3 g / 100 mL = 513 mEq/L

Administration
- Use infusion pump if available.
- Can be given via peripheral or central line.
- Use dedicated line if possible.
- Do not mix with other medications.

Example: 250 mL Bolus for ICP
- Give 2–5 mL/kg (Max 250 mL)
- Infuse over 10–20 minutes.

6. MONITORING

- Serum sodium every 2–4 hours
- Serum osmolality
- Neurological status / GCS
- Urine output
- Signs of fluid overload (edema, crackles, ↑ JVP)
- Vital signs continuously

Target sodium correction:
- 4–6 mEq/L in first 6 hours
- Do not exceed 8–10 mEq/L in 24 hours (risk of central pontine myelinolysis)

7. ADVERSE EFFECTS

Common
- Hypernatremia
- Hyperchloremic metabolic acidosis
- Nausea, vomiting
- Phlebitis (if peripheral line)

Serious
- Osmotic demyelination syndrome (central pontine myelinolysis)
- Pulmonary edema
- Congestive heart failure
- Renal impairment
- Seizures (rare)

⚠ Avoid rapid correction of sodium to prevent osmotic demyelination.

8. CALCULATION GUIDE

Sodium content in 3% Saline:

513 mEq Na^+ per liter
= 0.513 mEq/mL

Increase in Serum Sodium (Adrogué-Madias formula):

$$\Delta Na^+ = \frac{(\text{Infusate } Na^+ - \text{Serum } Na^+)}{\text{Total Body Water (L)} + 1}$$

Total Body Water (TBW)
- Men: 0.6 × body weight (kg)
- Women: 0.5 × body weight (kg)

9. IMPORTANT POINTS

- ✔ Use the lowest effective dose.
- ✔ Bolus therapy is for rapid reduction of ICP.
- ✔ In hyponatremia, correct slowly and cautiously.
- ✔ Stop infusion if Na^+ rising too quickly.
- ✔ Do not use in patients with fluid overload.
- ✔ Document exact time, dose, and sodium levels.
- ✔ Consult ICU/Nephrology for complex cases.

10. COMPATIBILITY / INCOMPATIBILITY

Compatible with:
- 0.9% Normal Saline

Do NOT mix with:
- Medications (use separate line)
- Dextrose solutions
- Blood products

Flush line with 0.9% NS before and after.

11. STORAGE

- Store at room temperature (15–30°C).
- Protect from light.
- Do not freeze.
- Use within 24 hours after opening.

12. KEY POINTS

- ✔ 3% saline reduces ICP by drawing water out of brain.
- ✔ Works within 5–15 minutes.
- ✔ Monitor sodium closely.
- ✔ Avoid overcorrection (> 8–10 mEq/L in 24 hr).
- ✔ Essential drug in neurocritical emergencies.

13. QUICK REFERENCE DOSE TABLE

INDICATION	BOLUS DOSE	INFUSION DOSE	NOTES
Raised ICP (Adults)	2–5 mL/kg IV over 10–20 min (Max 250 mL)	Repeat bolus if needed or per ICP	Assess clinically / ICP
Raised ICP (Pediatrics)	2–5 mL/kg IV over 10–20 min (Max 250 mL)	Repeat based on response	Use with caution
Symptomatic Hyponatremia (Adults)	100 mL IV over 10 min (may repeat up to 3 times)	0.5–1 mL/kg/hr	↑ Na^+ by 4–6 mEq/L in first 6 hr
Symptomatic Hyponatremia (Pediatrics)	2–5 mL/kg IV over 10–20 min	0.5–1 mL/kg/hr	Do not exceed 8–10 mEq/L in 24 hr

14. REMEMBER

RIGHT DRUG
RIGHT DOSE
RIGHT ROUTE
RIGHT TIME
SAVE THE BRAIN
SAVE LIVES

⚠ CORRECT INDICATION • CORRECT DOSE • CLOSE MONITORING • SAFE OUTCOMES

ALCOHOL WITHDRAWAL & DELIRIUM TREMENS
MANAGEMENT PROTOCOL

EARLY RECOGNITION • PROMPT TREATMENT • PREVENT COMPLICATIONS • SAVE LIVES

1. ASSESSMENT

- History of chronic alcohol use
- Last drink (time)
- Previous withdrawal / DT / seizures
- Comorbid illness / medications
- Physical examination
- Assess severity (use CIWA-Ar score)
- Exclude other causes of agitation / altered sensorium

2. ASSESS SEVERITY (CIWA-Ar)

SCORE	WITHDRAWAL SEVERITY
0 – 9	Mild
10 – 18	Moderate
19 – 30	Severe
> 30	Very severe / Impending DT

CIWA-Ar ≥ 15 = Severe withdrawal
CIWA-Ar ≥ 20 = High risk for DT

3. CLINICAL SPECTRUM & TIMELINE

6–12 h	Anxiety, tremor, sweating, insomnia, nausea
12–24 h	↑↑ symptoms, tachycardia, hypertension
24–48 h	Hallucinations, agitation, confusion, seizures
48–96 h	**Delirium Tremens** (autonomic instability, severe agitation, fever, delirium)

4. MANAGEMENT – ABCD APPROACH

A. STABILIZE (ABC)

- Airway – protect if GCS < 8 or severe agitation
- Breathing – give oxygen
- Circulation – IV access, monitor BP, HR, SpO_2
- Cardiac monitor
- Check RBS, temperature

B. INVESTIGATIONS

- CBC, RFT, LFT
- Serum electrolytes (Na^+, K^+, Mg^{2+})
- RBS
- ECG
- ABG (if indicated)
- Toxicology screen (if required)
- Others as per clinical condition

C. GENERAL MEASURES

- Quiet, dimly lit room
- Reassurance and reorientation
- IV fluids – NS / RL
- Correct dehydration
- Avoid physical restraints
- One-to-one nursing if severe agitation

D. SPECIFIC TREATMENT

- Benzodiazepines – mainstay
- **Thiamine before glucose**
- Correct electrolytes
- Symptomatic medications
- Treat complications

E. BENZODIAZEPINE THERAPY (TITRATE TO SYMPTOMS)

Symptom Triggered (Preferred) (Use CIWA-Ar score)

- CIWA-Ar < 10 : No medication
- CIWA-Ar 10–18 : Diazepam 10 mg IV/PO
- CIWA-Ar 19–30 : Diazepam 10–20 mg IV/PO
- CIWA-Ar > 30 : Diazepam 20 mg IV and repeat q 30–60 min until controlled

Fixed Schedule (Alternative)

- Diazepam 10 mg IV/PO 6th hourly

or

- Lorazepam 2–4 mg IV 6th hourly (use in elderly / liver disease)
- Taper gradually over 3–5 days

★ Diazepam is preferred (long acting).
Lorazepam preferred in liver disease / elderly.

F. ADJUNCTIVE THERAPY

Indication	Drug & Dose
Thiamine (Wernicke prophylaxis)	Thiamine 100 mg IV BD – 3 days then 100 mg PO OD
Electrolyte Correction	• $MgSO_4$ 1–2 g IV if low • KCl as per requirement • Correct Na^+
Agitation / Psychosis	Haloperidol 1–2 mg IV/PO 8th–12th hourly (if needed) (Avoid in severe DT unless necessary)
Seizures	Diazepam 10 mg IV stat (repeat if required)
Autonomic Hyperactivity	Clonidine 0.1–0.2 mg PO 8th hourly or Propranolol 10–20 mg PO 8th hourly (if no contraindication)
Nausea / Vomiting	Ondansetron 4 mg IV 8th hourly

G. DELIRIUM TREMENS (SEVERE WITHDRAWAL)

- CIWA-Ar ≥ 20 with confusion / hallucinations
- Fever, tachycardia, hypertension
- Profuse sweating, severe agitation
- +/- Seizures

- Manage in ICU / HDU
- High-dose benzodiazepines
- Aggressive hydration
- Correct electrolytes
- Monitor vitals, SpO_2, urine output
- Treat complications

H. MONITORING

PARAMETER	FREQUENCY / TARGET
CIWA-Ar score	2–4 hourly
Vital signs (HR, BP, RR, SpO_2)	Continuous / 2–4 hourly
Sedation level (RASS)	2–4 hourly (ICU)
Electrolytes	Daily
Fluid balance	Strict input / output
Blood glucose	4–6 hourly

RED FLAGS – ESCALATE CARE / ICU

- Refractory agitation despite medication
- Recurrent / prolonged seizures
- Severe autonomic instability
- Hyperthermia > 38.5°C
- Aspiration risk / respiratory compromise
- Hypotension not responding to fluids
- Need for continuous sedation or airway protection

I. COMPLICATIONS – BE ALERT

- Seizures
- Aspiration pneumonia
- Arrhythmias
- Acute coronary syndrome
- Electrolyte imbalance
- Wernicke encephalopathy
- Multiorgan dysfunction

Any complication → Escalate care / ICU

J. DISCHARGE CRITERIA

- CIWA-Ar < 10 for 24 hrs
- Stable vitals
- Oriented, calm, ambulatory
- Tolerating oral feeds
- Adequate family support / follow-up

K. PREVENTION OF RELAPSE

- Brief counselling
- Motivational therapy
- Refer to de-addiction services
- Pharmacotherapy (as indicated):
  - Acamprosate
  - Naltrexone
  - Disulfiram

L. KEY POINTS

- Benzodiazepines are the cornerstone.
- **Thiamine before glucose.**
- Treat the patient, not just the symptoms.
- Prevention of DT is better than treatment.
- Early recognition saves lives.

REFRACTORY DT – CONSIDER (IN ICU)

- Phenobarbital loading and infusion
- Dexmedetomidine infusion
- Propofol infusion (if intubated)
- Ketamine (adjunct in refractory cases)

TIMELINE AT A GLANCE

6–12 h	12–24 h	24–48 h	48–96 h
Tremor, anxiety, sweating	↑↑ Symptoms, tachycardia	Hallucinations, seizures	Delirium Tremens

NOTE: Protocol to be individualized as per patient condition and comorbidities.

www.ingramcontent.com/pod-product-compliance
Ingram Content Group UK Ltd.
Pitfield, Milton Keynes, MK11 3LW, UK
UKHW060019051026
15591UKWH00003B/275
* 9 7 9 8 9 0 5 6 0 1 6 2 0 *